Rosen's Management of Labor

Physician's Judgment and Patient Care

Second Edition

Edited by

Ralph Hale, M.D., F.A.C.O.G

Executive Director
The American College of Obstetricians and Gynecologists
Washington, DC

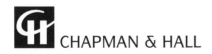

CHAPMAN & HALL

I ⓉP® **International Thomson Publishing**
Thomson Science

New York • Albany • Bonn • Boston • Cincinnati • Detroit • London • Madrid • Melbourne
Mexico City • Pacific Grove • Paris • San Francisco • Singapore • Tokyo • Toronto • Washington

Cover Design: Andrea Meyer, Emdash inc.

Copyright © 1998
Chapman & Hall

Printed in the United States of America

For more information, contact:

Chapman & Hall
115 Fifth Avenue
New York, NY 10003

Chapman & Hall
2-6 Boundary Row
London SE1 8HN
England

Thomas Nelson Australia
102 Dodds Street
South Melbourne, 3205
Victoria, Australia

Chapman & Hall GmbH
Postfach 100 263
D-69442 Weinheim
Germany

International Thomson Editores
Campos Eliseos 385, Piso 7
Col. Polanco
11560 Mexico D.F.
Mexico

International Thomson Publishing-Japan
Hirakawacho-cho Kyowa Building, 3F
1-2-1 Hirakawacho-cho
Chiyoda-ku, 102 Tokyo
Japan

International Thomson Publishing Asia
221 Henderson Road #05-10
Henderson Building
Singapore 0315

1 2 3 4 5 6 7 8 9 10 XXX 01 00 99 98

Library of Congress Cataloging-in-Publication Data

Rosen's management of labor : physician's judgment and patient care /
    editor, Ralph W. Hale. —2nd ed.
      p.   cm.
    Rev. ed. of: Management of labor / Mortimer G. Rosen. c1990.
    Includes bibliographical references and index.
    ISBN 0-412-13811-5 (alk. paper)
    1. Labor (Obstetrics). I. Labor (Obstetrics)—Complications. 3. Obstetrics—Descision
    making. I. Hale, Ralph W., 1935-   . II. Rosen, Mortimer G. Management of labor.
      [DNLM: 1. Labor. 2. Delivery. 3. Judgment. WQ 300 R8135 1997]
    RG651.R67   1997   618.4—dc21   DNLM/DLC
    for Library of Congress   97-3650
                                                     CIP

British Library Cataloguing in Publication Data available

To order this or any other Chapman & Hall book, please contact **International Thomson Publishing, 7625 Empire Drive, Florence, KY 41042.** Phone: (606) 525-6600 or 1-800-842-3636.
Fax: (606) 525-7778, e-mail: order@chaphall.com.

For a complete listing of Chapman & Hall's titles, send your requests to
Chapman & Hall, Dept. BC, 115 Fifth Avenue, New York, NY 10003.

*This book is dedicated to
the clinician who applies the art of obstetrics
to the care of two patients during labor,
and who promises the best judgment,
but cannot guarantee a perfect outcome.*

Contents

Preface 1st edition

Dr. Mortimer Rosen

Medical care is often not limited to a single treatment. At the bedside several options for patient care may be present. The selection of the best treatment option, in large part, involves judgment. The use of good judgment, to the best of his or her ability, is explicit in the physician's oath. However, judgment is fallible. Therefore, a perfect outcome is always a goal to be sought, but not always an outcome which can be reached.

There are several purposes in this clinical text, the first of which is to present standard definitions or a dictionary of terms so that a common language may be used with universal understanding. Then, options for clinical choices that describe a philosophy for labor management will be presented. Labor management always involves several clinical choices.

If all obstetricians were to use the same definitions to describe the events of labor, this would lead to better understanding of all obstetrical practices. The standard set of definitions would simplify outcome comparisons between the several choices in medical practice. In turn, the ability to compare results would lead to more reasoned methods for improved clinical care.

In this text, definitions will be presented so that all clinicians will speak the same language. For instance, the word *dystocia* has little meaning. Chapter 9 is dedicated to reviewing the many uses of this word and the resulting confusion this term causes. Replace *dystocia* with the phrase *arrest in active phase labor* that can be defined, understood, measured, and conveys more meaning.

In presenting protocols for patient care in this text, when complete information is lacking, it will be noted. For example, except in the most indirect manner, the electronic fetal heart monitor does not evaluate the brain and cannot provide direct information about fetal brain damage. Monitoring devices display fetal heart rate data and maternal uterine contraction activity that relate to fetal risk and potential for acidosis. The link to damage occurring in the brain at the time of monitoring cannot be made.

When more than one clinical choice is present, the several choices will be described. It is apparent that clinical care often involves several choices. Therefore, absolutes or rules are often limiting. Absolutes omit the art of judgment, and in individual patient care situations absolute rules rarely are appropriate. Guidelines suggest flexibility and allow more latitude.

If obstetricians cannot maintain the art of patient care, then the art may soon disappear. Obstetrical care will be diminished by the loss of decision choices and judgment. It is important that attention be paid to certain realities in this specialty. The vaginal birth route is not the alternative birth route. The correct cesarean birth rate is not known. The key for the clinician is choice followed by a judgment that is based on what is known.

This book is not written to replace standard texts, nor is it meant to serve as an encyclopedia of information. Rather, it represents a philosophy of and guidelines to patient care.

Preface, 2nd edition

This book was originally written by Mortimer Rosen, MD, the Willard C. Rappleye Professor and Chair of the Department of Obstetrics and Gynecology at the College of Physicians and Surgeons of Columbia University, as well as Director of Obstetrics and Gynecology at Sloane Hospital for Women. Dr. Rosen was an outstanding practitioner and teacher of the science, as well as the art, of obstetrics. He was recognized by his peers and the American College of Obstetricians and Gynecologists for his outstanding contributions to the specialty. In 1991 Dr. Rosen was given the Outstanding District Service Award in recognition of his activities. Dr. Rosen died in 1992.

Dr. Rosen published many articles, books, chapters, and other work during his career. One of these was the current book, *Management of Labor*. This was a topic that Dr. Rosen felt very important to obstetrics, and he was concerned that future generations of obstetricians would lose the skill of clinical management and rely instead on technology. For Dr. Rosen the close association between the physician and patient was essential; he knew that clinical management on a personal level was essential to the relationship. Some might say this is old-fashioned medicine, but others, like Dr. Rosen, maintain that the art of patient care forms the core of being an obstetrician.

We are thankful that Dr. Lynn Rosen, Dr. Mortimer Rosen's wife, has allowed the American College of Obstetricians and Gynecologist the opportunity to continue the publication of this book. As Dr. Rosen so aptly stated in his preface to the first edition, which follows, "this book . . . represents a philosophy of and guideline to patient care. The key for the clinician is choice followed by a judgment based on what is known."

In keeping with his original thoughts and philosophy, Dr. Rosen's original writing has been maintained and only edited to reflect changes that have occurred in the 6 years since the original publication. ACOG Educational Bulletins, Committee Opinions, and Practice Patterns have also been utilized as appropriate to reinforce current concepts and to present additional ideas. Several new chapters have been added to further enhance the book, and some of the original chapters have been combined for a better presentation. However, in all instances the original philosophy of Dr. Rosen has been maintained. The ability of the obstetrician to evaluate a patient and make a judgment for the management of the patient based on this evaluation is essential. The ability to evaluate and determine the choice among options in medicine is, and must always remain, the right of the physician.

I would also like to extend my thanks to Ms. Terrie Gibson for the numerous hours she spent typing this manuscript. Without her effort, this edition would not have been possible.

Contributors

Ann Allen, JD, Corporate Counsel and Director of Legal Affairs, American College of Obstetricians and Gynecologists

Larry P. Griffin, MD, Director of Program Services, American College of Obstetricians and Gynecologists

Ralph W. Hale, MD, Executive Director, American College of Obstetricians and Gynecologists

Ken Heland, JD, Associate Director of Program Services, American College of Obstetricians and Gynecologists

Gerald Holzman, MD, Director of Education, American College of Obstetricians and Gynecologists

Stanley Zinberg, MD, Director of Practice Activities, American College of Obstetricians and Gynecologists

Chapter 1

Understanding Morbidity and Mortality in the Management of Labor

Overview

The Crisis

Today there is great confusion in obstetrical practice concerning the effect of medical interventions during labor on infant outcome. This confusion has resulted in dramatic changes in obstetrical practice in an effort to decrease the likelihood of a poor outcome, often with little or no objective evidence that a specific change will effect produce an improvement. This is illustrated by the significant increases in cesarean birthrate in an attempt to lower infant morbidity and mortality.

In 1984, the estimated total cesarean birthrate was about 21.2%. In 1987, the estimated cesarean rate rose to 25%.[1] By 1994 the rates in some facilities were above 30%.[2] In order to justify the rising use of such an operative intervention, maternal and perinatal morbidity and mortality reviews should document a continuing improvement in maternal and fetal outcomes that correspond to the rising cesarean birthrate; this has not occurred.

Although remarkable decreases in death and damage to mother and fetus have taken place during the past 30 years, the maternal and fetal improvements in outcome are not directly related to the cesarean birthrate. Most cesareans are performed in healthy women at term. The quality of obstetrical, care far transcends the cesarean birth. It is this type of assumed, but inaccurate, cause-and-effect relationship, as well as the external forces of patients and society, that confront the physician and have helped to create confusion in clinical practice. The crisis is that continuing intervention is not leading to continuing improvement in maternal and fetal outcome. In fact, intervention may be associated not only with no improvement in outcome, but also with increased risk of injury to mother or newborn. Additionally, the increased costs of many interventions divert limited health resources away from services of proven benefit to those that are, at best, uncertain. Possibly even worse is the fact that the false belief that any such intervention may be of benefit may delay finding the real cause of a poor outcome and either working toward its prevention or, at the least, avoiding the very real legal risks to the public, or having the legal profession believe that the cause of a poor outcome was not using such an unproven approach.

Objectives

At the conclusion of this chapter, the clinician should understand the relationships among the following:

1. Cesarean delivery and patient outcome
2. Maternal risk and obstetrical intervention
3. Fetal risk and obstetrical intervention
4. Patients' expectations and their influences on care
5. Fear of litigation and its influence on obstetrical intervention

Maternal Mortality Rates

For many years maternal mortality conferences were a part of every hospital's teaching program. They greatly helped clinicians as they sought better under-standing of and new methods for avoiding maternal deaths by allowing them to learn from their colleagues' management experiences. In the 20th century mater-nal mortality has continued to decrease. In 1935 the maternal mortality rate was 582 per 100,000 live births; it had fallen to 8.3 per 100,000 live births by 1994. During 1994 leading causes of maternal mortality were hypertensive disorders of pregnancy, hemorrhage, infections, and embolism.[3,4]

Deaths have become so infrequent that maternal mortality conferences have fallen largely into disuse. Conferences related to maternal and fetal medical com-plications during pregnancy have replaced mortality as the criteria for conference case selections.

As an example of this changing focus of obstetrics, during 1982 in the city of Philadelphia only one citywide maternal mortality conference was held, and that conference was held only at the insistence of an interested physician who had recently moved to Philadelphia. No citywide maternal mortality conference was held in the next several years. Today, although the classic etiologies for maternal deaths—hemorrhage, infection, and toxemia—are still present and important, they are being challenged by new maternal risk factors, such as obstetrical com-plications involving cesarean surgery and, increasingly, HIV infection.

Maternal Mortality Due to Cesarean

Despite the fact that one Boston hospital could record more than 10,000 cesarean births without an operative-related maternal death, any use of anesthesia, no matter how expertly given, is associated with an increased risk of both morbidity and mortality. In addition, although anesthetic care is generally at a high level of safety, its availability, the quality and expertise of the anesthetist, and the range of options varies both with hospital size and the number of obstetrical deliveries.

Causes of maternal morbidity following cesarean include infection, estimated to be between 20% and 30%,[7] which exceeds the rate for maternal infections following spontaneous birth.[6] In today's rapidly changing epidemiology of infection, the introduction of HIV/AIDS add new potential risk factors. It is not unusual for a patient to tell her obstetrician that she fears infection, with HIV or other agents, by blood transfusion, which is an increased risk following cesarean surgery. In reality, the risk of these transmissions following transfusion of properly screened blood is remote, but it is increased when compared with no such risk. The average blood loss following cesarean birth may exceed 1000 ml and is two to three times higher than blood loss following spontaneous vaginal birth.[8]

Review of available data documents maternal mortality following emergency cesarean being twice the rate of maternal mortality following spontaneous birth.[9] Some of this increase in morbidity and mortality is a result of the clinical condition associated with the indications for the cesarean itself. Even elective cesarean results in a twofold increase in maternal deaths. Thus, while the cesarean is an extremely low-risk procedure, it is associated with increased maternal morbidity and mortality when compared with vaginal delivery.

The maternal data may be summarized by noting that the actual surgical risks for maternal death are extremely low and have been remarkably improved through better understanding of surgical technique, anesthetic use, blood transfusion, and prevention and treatment of infection. Yet the many inherent forms of morbidity in this procedure do not support the statement sometimes made that there is little difference in maternal risk between vaginal birth and cesarean birth.

Fetal Risk Replaces Maternal Risk

Fetal care often seems to dominate maternal care as our primary focus in contemporary obstetrics. As noted, because maternal risk from cesarean is small, the clinical choice of cesarean is far easier and allows greater freedom of choice when considering more complicated vaginal birth events and obstetric operations, such as the breech birth, delivery of twins, and use of obstetrical midforceps. The driving force behind most clinical decisions during labor today is concern for the quality of life of the fetus. Avoiding intrapartum CNS damage is a high priority. Because of its influence on patient care, infant CNS deficit is addressed in Chapter 2; this is an important issue. The prevalence of cerebral palsy from all causes is today estimated to be between one and three affected children per 1000 children at 7 to 20 years of age, with one half of those following premature birth.

Perinatal mortality has continued to decrease, and this change suggests an improvement in fetal and neonatal therapy as well as advances in obstetric management. Less clear is what specific factors contribute most to these improved infant outcomes. For example, in New York state from 1968 to 1977, perinatal mortality rates fell and cesarean birthrates increased almost in parallel. This could suggest a related effect of the rising cesarean birthrate on infant outcome. However, if the second half of this time period alone is examined, the cesarean birthrate continued to increase, but the perinatal mortality rates decreased much more slowly. This obviously makes the idea of a cause-and-effect relationship between more cesareans and improved infant outcome a tenuous concept.

As we approach the goal of lowered risk and morbidity, the size of the high-risk target population becomes smaller; therefore, the identification of the at-risk fetus becomes more difficult. Today a large percentage of the fetal-risk population lies in the under 1500 g low-birthweight group. This low-birthweight group probably contributes to more than 75% of perinatal mortality, although the low-birthweight population (less than 2500 g) accounts for less than 5% to 12% of all births. Operative intervention as the major method for improving infant outcome would not remove all or even most causes of CNS deficits or infant morbidity in this low-birthweight population. The answer to the question of how many cesareans are justified to approach our goals of diminished maternal and perinatal morbidity is not clear. It is clear that attempting to eliminate or even reduce the risk of cerebral palsy by cesarean section has not been successful.[10,11]

Patient Expectations of a Perfect Outcome and Malpractice Accusations

Complicating the treatment choices during labor are patient expectations of a perfect outcome. Anything less than a healthy infant raises the question, Why did the morbidity occur? The clinician's judgment and medical decisions are complicated by the fear of malpractice accusations and the associated emotional and financial risks.

There are few practicing obstetricians who have not been queried or deposed by a plaintiff's attorney. According to the American College of Obstetricians and Gynecologists (ACOG), 79.4% of ACOG Fellows have been sued once and 58% have been sued more than once.[12] All obstetricians know of associates who have been sued in poor-outcome situations. The physician's personal distress may be so profound that even when the clinician originally believed that the patient care was correct, by the end of a deposition or trial, or after many months of reevaluation, both in public and in private, personal doubts may created. For that physician the safer choice the "next time" may be an attempt to reach a "lower risk" personal situation sooner. In these cases, the decision to do a cesarean is usually made. Almost all published reports indicate cesarean birthrates are higher in private practice environments than among the non–private practice population, despite the fact that the latter population is at higher medical risk.

To the obstetrician practicing in this arena, four theories of the relationship between patient care and malpractice risk are offered:

1. If you practice good obstetrics and maternal and infant outcomes are good, you are unlikely to be sued.
2. If you practice poor obstetrics (not recommended) and maternal and fetal outcomes are good, you are unlikely to be sued.
3. If you practice good obstetrics and either maternal or fetal outcome is poor, you are likely to be sued.
4. If you practice poor obstetrics and either maternal or fetal outcome is poor, you are likely to be sued.

Therefore, if you are to be sued on the basis of clinical outcome, not on the basis of clinical care, why not practice good obstetrics? (This is not to say that the clinical care given is unimportant in a legal sense.) In fact, excellent, well-recorded documents can often prevent a lawsuit from being pursued even after an initial malpractice claim has been filed.

Summary

1. Changes of medical practice in obstetrics must be justified by improving outcome for mother and fetus, especially should its changes pose additional risks or costs.
2. Morbidity and mortality rates for both neonate and mother have improved markedly during the 20th century. The rise in cesarean birth during the past 15 years cannot easily be casually linked with the decrease in morbidity.
3. The cesarean, a relatively safe procedure, carries increased risk for the mother in both present and future pregnancies.
4. The cesarean may be a safe birth route for the fetus of the present pregnancy but carries increased risk for the fetus of a future otherwise uncomplicated pregnancy.

References

1. Shiono PH, Fielden JG, McNellis D, et al. Recent trends in cesarean birth and trial of labor rates in the U.S. JAMA 1987;257:494–497.
2. Lagrew DC, Morgan MA. Decreasing the cesarean section rate in a private hospital: Success without mandated clinical changes. Am J Obstet Gynecol 1996;174: 184–191.

3. Center for Disease Control and Prevention, Monthly Vital Statistics Report. 1996, 45(Suppl).

4. Berg CJ, Afrash HK, Koonin LM, Tucker M. Pregnancy related mortality in the United States, 1987–90. Obstet Gynecol 1996;88:161–167.

5. Schneider J. Personal communication 1982.

6. Shiono PH, McNellis DM, Rhoads GG. Reasons for the rising cesarean delivery rates; 1978–1984. Obstet Gynecol 1987;69:696–700.

7. Beattie PG, Ping TR, Hunter MF, Lake Y. Risk factors for wound infection following cesarean section. Aust N Z J Obstet Gynecol 1994;34:398–402.

8. Pritchard JA, MacDonald PC, Grant N. Williams Obstetrics, ed 17. Norwalk, CT, Appleton-Century-Crofts, 1985, pp 3, 193, 356.

9. Miller JM. Maternal and neonatal morbidity and mortality in cesarean section. Obstet Gynecol Clinics North Am 1988;15:629–638.

10. ACOG. Fetal and Neonatal Neurologic Injury: American College of Obstetricians and Gynecologists Technical Bulletin #163, 1992. Washington, DC, ACOG.

11. Australian and New Zealand Perinatal Society. Consensus statement of the origins of cerebral palsy. Med J Aust 1995;162:85–89.

12. ACOG Professional Liability Survey 1992. Washington, DC, ACOG.

Chapter 2

Infant Neurologic Deficiency: Linkage with Labor

Overview

In this chapter and throughout the book, the term *brain damage* will not be used often. It falsely implies that in all cases of neurologic deficit, the brain was once normal and then damaged. Since such differences are often the result of abnormal development of a brain that was not normal to begin with, we use the more generic terms *neurologic* or *CNS deficit.* In the introduction it was noted that one of the forces modulating the changing clinical care of women during labor was the concern, of both the physician and patient, with the later appearance of an infant brain deficit. This infant pathology is often defined in terms of three major categories: mental retardation, epilepsy, and cerebral palsy. Although there are many other forms of brain dysfunction, such as behavioral problems and learning disorders, these have not been etiologically attributed to events in the intrapartal period.

These three major neurologic categories—cerebral palsy, epilepsy, and mental retardation—are discussed as distinct and separate entities. Cerebral palsy is a nonprogressive motor dysfunction that may or may not include mental retardation and convulsions. It is an illness that differs from pure epilepsy and pure mental retardation.

In this chapter the pathophysiologies of developmental brain injury and deficiencies are reviewed. If a relationship has been identified that links these conditions to events occurring in labor, it is discussed. Attention is directed to the association of fetal distress, fetal acidosis, and Apgar scores with neurologic difficulties. For a more complete review of prenatal and perinatal events as they relate to brain damage, the reader is referred to the review entitled *Prenatal and Perinatal Factors Associated with Brain Disorders* published in 1985 by the National Institute of Health[1] and summarized in a later review article.[2]

Objectives

At the conclusion of this chapter, the clinician should understand the following:

1. Pathologic findings associated with infant CNS deficiency
2. Neurologic deficiency syndromes associated with obstetrical care
3. Relationships between CNS deficiencies and
    a. Intrapartal asphyxia
    b. Apgar scores
    c. Birth route
    d. Fetal distress

Pathophysiology of Hypoxia-Related Brain Damage

Reasons for Confusion

The causes for the death of brain cells in the fetal and neonatal brain are still unclear. In the vast majority of cases of neurologic deficiencies, there is no casual relationship to obstetric management. In the small number that relate to obstetrical interventions during labor, gross neurologic injuries may be divided into those associated with hypoxia and, less frequently, those injuries associated with direct fetal trauma.

Other clinical problems, such as infection or genetic defects, are not included in this review. The term *asphyxia* is often applied, but it is identified with poorly understood modifiers such as acute or chronic asphyxia, or perinatal, neonatal, or intrapartal asphyxia. Since asphyxia implies total lack of oxygen, it is difficult to define the event. Related terms may identify a length of time or a period of life, but they remain vague. For example, the term *perinatal asphyxia* may extend from 28 weeks of fetal life to 28 days of neonatal life. This term adds little information as to when an insult to the brain may have occurred. It does not give us a day of injury or a cause for the damage. It merely describes a long period of time during which an event may have occurred.

The words *anoxia* and *asphyxia* may be well defined in textbooks but unfortunately are not used with precision in the clinical arena. Certainly there is risk for brain damage with prolonged asphyxia or anoxia if either occurs. How much oxygen deficit must be present before brain damage occurs, or what other factors may increase the fetal and neonatal risk for actual damage, are not well understood. Unfortunately, the use of these terms implies that damage will or has occurred, and that is usually an incorrect assumption. On the other hand, *hypoxia* is a more accurate description of the event usually seen in clinical practice. By definition, hypoxia implies some reduction of oxygenation but not a total lack of oxygen. As such, the term has a less ominous impression. This allows the obstetrician and pediatrician to evaluate the outcome and describe the length and degree of the *hypoxia episode*. Hypoxia does not imply brain damage, especially when rapidly corrected. *Asphyxia* should never appear in the medical record.

Infant Brain Damage

EXAMPLE OF FETAL NUTRIENT SUPPLY RISK CONFOUNDED BY PREMATURITY AND LABOR

Long-standing, poor placental nutrient (including oxygen) supply in a chronic hypertensive mother was associated with a severely growth-retarded fetus at labor onset at 32 weeks of gestation. Onset-of-labor monitoring revealed late fetal heart-rate decelerations.

Comment

The preexisting supply problem may be a greater risk for morbidity than the acute fetal supply problem during labor, as suggested by the late decelerations. There is no clinical information separating the acute from the chronic events. In addition, the same degree of uteroplacental insufficiency in the term fetus may result in different effects from those that occur in the very low-birthweight fetus, as occurred in this example. If later neurologic deficits are diagnosed, it is more likely that they were caused by events before labor even began.

The term *may* is used cautiously. Immaturity has generally been spoken of as a time of greater resistance to cell death when compared with older organisms. However, problems such as intracerebral hemorrhage occur more often at the lowest birthweights and are associated with increased risk of neurologic deficits. It is known that the immature brain is more sensitive to hypoxia than the more mature. In these examples, deprivation of fetal supply is inferred.

Should the obstetrician intervene? Will intervention decrease fetal risks?

EXAMPLE OF ABNORMAL LABOR CONFOUNDED BY AN ABNORMAL FETAL HEART-RATE PATTERN

A term mother undergoes an arrest in the active phase of labor followed by a series of deep, variable decelerations as she enters the second stage of labor. Is her fetus more vulnerable to brain damage following a series of variable fetal heart-rate decelerations than a fetus facing variable decelerations during a normal active-phase labor?

Comment

Confounding factors such as these raise obvious questions, but the answers to these questions are not known. The two problems may be additive or they may add no increased risk, yet the obstetrician more often intervenes in the face of two abnormalities than when faced with only one. The diagnosis of dystocia with a non-reassuring fetal heart-rate pattern is a frequent one. The risk for neurologic damage in the presence of dystocia is quite low and is described more completely in Chapter 9.

Neuropathology of Neurologic Deficit Associated with Asphyxia

The early potential endpoints of the problems of perinatal hypoxia may be seen by the clinician as intracranial bleeding and edema. The potential endpoints, after these acute events, are visualized as nerve death, gross CNS morphologic change, and altered neurologic function of the child. However, it must be mentioned that even when the early signs of so-called hypoxia injury are seen, the evolution from these early signs to later abnormal development and function cannot be predicted with significant accuracy.

EXAMPLE OF EVOLUTION OF NEUROPATHOLOGIC EVENTS

In a term fetus, a prolonged compression of the umbilical cord was associated with the birth of a severely depressed, Apgar 2 and 4, infant. Cerebral edema, and subarachnoid and intraventricular hemorrhage, were later visualized on ultrasonographic studies during the first several days of life. Clinical signs of neurologic dysfunction were seen during the first 12 hours. Seizures occurred during the next several days. At the time of discharge the neonate appeared to be feeding well, and the seizures were controlled by medication. During the neonatal period, reliable prediction of future development abnormalities was not possible, but the prognosis was guarded at the time of discharge.

Comment

Unfortunately, because of the likely cell death in the baby's brain, this neonate, who had been normocephalic at birth, was microcephalic 1 year later. By that time the clinical picture was certain, and the child did have later cognitive and motor pathology.

Note: This does not mean that all or even most clinical situations can be linked to peripartum events. The injurious insult could have occurred prior to the onset of labor but was not diagnosable until labor began.

To describe this pathology, broad classifications, which include hemorrhage and edema, are used. In the case of fetal and neonatal CNS bleeding, there are three general categories of bleeding: subdural, subarachnoid, and intracerebral. For purposes of simplifying this discussion, the cephalhematoma, or extracranial bleed, which often occurs spontaneously or in association with trauma, very rarely causes brain damage and will not be described or discussed.

Subdural Hemorrhage

The subdural bleed, or subdural hematoma, is a lesion that is relatively uncommon in current obstetrical practice because of the trend to avoid traumatic labors and deliveries. During the last 25 years, the practice of obstetrics has turned away from the use of the high or difficult midforceps, or the acceptance of excessively prolonged labors. Thus, this category, once prominent, is now uncommon.

In association with a subdural bleed there are lacerations of the larger veins of the *dura* mater. When the subdural hemorrhage occurs, it is seen in the term fetus more frequently than in the low-birthweight fetus and is often associated with physical trauma to the fetal head. The classic clinical picture associated with this pathology occurs in a patient who has had a difficult forceps application following a protraction or arrest in the active phase of labor, or following a delay in the descent of the vertex. The hematoma, or bleed, may be associated with a skull fracture, but usually this is not present. It should be noted that the trauma that causes a subdural bleed can occur in either labor or delivery. It should not be inferred that the trauma in such a case was necessarily due to a forceps delivery. In fact, in cases of a nondifficult forceps application and delivery, it is likely that the forceps operation may have prevented further ongoing trauma. The neonate often becomes depressed shortly after birth, and as the neonate recovers from the trauma, he or she begins to display signs of abnormal neurologic function, such as changes in muscle tone, irritability, and seizures. This subdural hemorrhage is frequently associated with severe infant developmental pathology, such as cerebral palsy, with motor and cognitive dysfunction.

Subarachnoid Hemorrhage

This type of intracranial bleed is more frequently seen than the subdural hemorrhage. This hemorrhage may be isolated to the subarachnoid space, or it may be seen in association with intracerebral bleeding. Although on occasion subarachnoid bleeding may be associated with trauma, it is usually found in association with clinical signs of fetal distress that precipitated the potentially traumatic intervention in the first place.

Most subarachnoid hemorrhages are diagnosed in the neonate and are often associated with clinical risk conditions such as fetal acidosis or hypoxia. Perhaps three quarters of all subarachnoid hemorrhages are seen in the lowest birthweight neonates, with the remaining 25% being seen in term infants. It should be noted that these bleeds are also be found unassociated with known risks of labor.

The subarachnoid bleed usually relates to some form of fetal deprivation of supply. The term *hypoxia* is a more specific supply problem. These terms do not completely overlap. The expression *deprivation of supply* includes not only cell respiratory problems, such as hypoxia, but all metabolic problems, including nutritional deprivation, as seen in intrauterine growth retardation. Several confounding clinical events may be present and confuse the etiology of subarachnoid hemorrhage. It is not true that the pressure of a subarachnoid bleed is both evidence of and/or results from perinatal hypoxia.

EXAMPLE OF CONFOUNDING RISK FOR
SUBARACHNOID HEMORRHAGE

Intrapartum fetal distress occurred in a growth-deprived premature 1753-g infant. During the neonatal period, the infant had severe respiratory distress.

Comment

Which risks caused this infant's damage? The brain was already at risk because of the prenatal problem of growth retardation. This was confounded by preterm birth and non-reassuring fetal status on fetal monitoring. Later, the neonatal condition of respiratory distress occurred with the clinical risk associated neurologic deficit. Are these risks linked, cumulative, or independent? In individual cases, the answers to these questions are usually unclear.

Subarachnoid bleeding usually occurs during the immediate neonatal period, the time when most brain hemorrhage occurs. The confusion in the association of several risk factors makes it difficult to assign etiology in other than a general manner. All of these individual clinical conditions are risks for potential harm. Each of these conditions might increase the risk for subarachnoid bleeding. Initial causes for these problems are not easily documented. Stated differently, the presence of intrapartum fetal distress seen during electronic monitoring is likely to be a result of previously existing CNS deficiencies or could be signaling an acute problem that, if untreated, might increase the risk for brain dysfunction.

Intracerebral Hemorrhage

Although originally noted to take place around the cerebral ventricles and associated with a finding called *periventricular leukoencephalomalacia,* intracerebral bleeding also takes place away from the ventricles and within all areas of the brain. Intracerebral bleeding is most frequently associated with prematurity. The lowest birthweight fetuses (<1500 g) have the highest incidence of periventricular and intracerebral bleeding. We do not know how to avoid this injury. One clinical question, which is yet unanswered, is whether some of the physiologic problems of prematurity can be partially overcome by altering the fetal birth route. This raises the question of whether there is any birthweight below which cesarean delivery is the route of choice. Stated differently, is the physical pressure on the brain during vaginal birth an increased risk for intracerebral bleeding? Does hypoxia occur more often in low-birthweight fetuses because of an intolerance to labor?

The answer to the pathophysiology of these intracerebral hemorrhages may lie in the maturity of fetal blood vessels.[3] This has resulted in dramatic changes in obstetrical practice in an effort to decrease the likelihood of a poor outcome, often with little or no objective evidence that a specific change will effect such an improvement. The immature blood vessels in the developing brain of a low-birth-weight fetus or neonate are no more than several cells thick. When exposed to stress associated with hypoxia and acidosis, or pressure on the vertex, or both stresses, the intracerebral circulation changes and flow through the smaller blood vessels may stop as the blood pressure falls. Without blood flow, these thin-walled vessels may become damaged due to lack of supply. When circulation is restored, blood flows through these damaged vessels and intracerebral bleeding occurs.

Infant Brain Damage

This intracerebral hemorrhage is closely linked with fetal immaturity. Intracerebral bleeding can also occur in association with neonatal events such as continuous positive airway pressure and neonatal respiratory distress.

In the past the ability to diagnose cerebral edema was limited to its diagnosis on the basis of physical examination, primarily tenseness of the fontanels and increased spinal fluid pressure. It is much more easily and frequently found today with the availability and frequent use of computed tomography, magnetic resonance imaging, and ultrasonography. As a result, edema, which was often overlooked previously, is identified, and more information regarding cerebral edema has been made available.

Cerebral Edema

Cerebral edema occurs more frequently in the term infant than the preterm infant, usually in association with a difficult labor or fetal findings in labor that are non-reassuring. Although hemorrhage may also occur in term infants, as a general statement, bleeding is seen more frequently in the less mature fetus. Intracerebral edema represents a reaction to an injury and may be associated with cell necrosis. Depending on the severity of the events that lead to the edema, there may be varying degrees of both brain damage and risk for future abnormal brain development functions.

Association of Pathology with Function

Brain Plasticity

In all attempts to correlate pathology with later malfunction, several confounding problems must be considered. In the first, called *plasticity of the brain,* the brain may have sufficient reserve or new resources for compensating for whatever injury or damage has occurred. *Plasticity* implies the ability of a different area of the brain to take over a function for a damaged area. As a corollary, attempts to quantitate motor or cognitive effects of a potentially injurious event may be limited when the pathology is small and when an alternate area of the brain assumes or returns the lost function. The question of how many cells must be damaged before brain damage can be recognized is unanswerable. Each organ has a great deal of reserve function. The expression of and testing for intellectual, behavioral, or motor ability in the neonate or infant is limited. In the neonatal period there are no accepted useful clinical tests that, when given during the first few days of life, predict later intelligence or motor ability. A neonatal brain may be damaged and at risk for cerebral palsy, yet many months or even years may pass before cerebral palsy or other CNS defects are identified clinically.

Linkage of Specific Cerebral Pathology with Clinical Damage

As already noted, the presence of brain hemorrhage, or edema, is not always associated with neurologic damage. Why some infants adapt to the bleed and perform normally and yet, following the same clinical events, other infants are damaged is not clear. Even more confusing is the fact that the terms *perinatal asphyxia* and *asphyxia neonatorum* have been used in an attempt to identify the cause of many infant neurologic diseases extending from cerebral palsy through the learning disorders.[1] The inconsistent use of these terms, the lack of a universally acceptable definition, and the lack of a firm relationship between these diagnoses and later developments of CNS abnormalities has been and is a source of great concern.

Autopsy studies have found that the same intracerebral pathology does not always follow a single etiologic factor. Conversely, 28 different morphologic brain abnormalities have been attributed to the same clinical function or illness.[1] The problem may be diagrammed as follows:

CONFUSION IN UNDERSTANDING INFANT BRAIN DAMAGE

Same cerebral pathology is associated with many clinical forms of damage

Different clinical insults may result in a single area of brain damage

Different clinical events may result in perinatal asphyxia

Functional CNS pathology may be associated with many different forms of damage injury in the same area of the brain. The resultant clinical events may result in a similar clinical picture yet not be associated with the same etiology. This confusion in etiology leaves the clinician perplexed when trying to prevent morbidity. Patient care techniques must be chosen, often without adequate etiologic information.

Infant Brain Damage

Neurologic Damage, Fetal Risk, and Fetal Maturity

Another factor obscuring the link between fetal risk and infant outcome is the degree of fetal maturity at the time a clinical risk factor occurs. The dynamic fetal condition, rapidly changing and evolving from a less mature organism to a more mature organism in utero (or as a neonate), may in part explain the reasons for the confusion.

EXAMPLE OF SAME FETAL RISK OCCURRING AT DIFFERENT FETAL MATURITY STAGES, PRODUCING TWO DIFFERENT CLINICAL SYNDROMES CALLED *CEREBRAL PALSY*

The clinical findings of cerebral palsy that follows a fetal brain injury that took place at 28 weeks of maturity are different from the clinical findings of cerebral palsy following a brain injury that took place at 38 weeks of maturity. The infants have different motor and cognitive deficits when seen at 2 years of age. This indicates that different areas of the fetal brain have different levels of vulnerability to the same stimulus at different stages of development.

Comment

The low-birthweight fetus may hemorrhage in response to the effects of prolonged umbilical cord compression. In contrast, the term infant may display diffuse cortical edema in response to the same insult. Injuries that may result will occur in different parts of the brain. Both infants may express cerebral pathology but in different ways. The same clinical risk may lead to one clinical form of cerebral palsy in the low-birthweight fetus, and a different clinical form of cerebral palsy in the term fetus. Thus, the same high-risk event at different periods of human development leads to different forms of functional CNS deficit.

Avoiding Fetal Brain Damage

It is clear that brain injury may result from pathologic human development from the time of conception throughout the fetal period. In the majority of cases the clinician and patient have the intuitive feeling that brain damage can be avoided by obstetrical interventions in and around labor. This concept is too narrow and clearly erroneous.

As noted in a recent report from the National Institutes of Health, cytogenetic, biochemical, and teratogenic events, and many other intrauterine problems, such as deprivation of fetal nutrients and in utero fetal infections, are associated with a fetus that is already damaged or mentally retarded at the time of labor. This existing brain damage is unknown to the clinician because there are no reliable tests for in utero brain function.

EXAMPLE OF AN ALREADY DAMAGED FETUS NOT IMPROVED BY CESAREAN DELIVERY

If the breech presentation fetus is already brain damaged, that may be one of the reason it moves differently in utero and assumes the breech position.

Comment

Most fetuses in breech presentations are neurologically normal. However, the incidence of preexisting fetal brain damage in this population is higher than that for the vertex presentation group. Therefore, all breech presentations are already at higher risk for CNS morbidity than the vertex presentation of the same birthweight. This is true regardless of mode of delivery.

EXAMPLE OF AN ALREADY DAMAGED FETUS THAT MAY EXHIBIT INTRAPARTAL FETAL DISTRESS

The growth-retarded or postmature fetus with little metabolic reserve due to supply (nutrient) deprivation for the previous week will quickly show electronic monitoring signs of late decelerations when labor begins. Was brain damage present or did labor cause brain damage?

Comment

It is impossible to consistently identify this damaged brain prior to birth. If this fetus is already damaged, it might react abnormally to labor and present with non-reassuring fetal heart patterns. The best clinical example is the fetal heart-rate monitoring tracing in which there is absence of beat-to-beat variability when the fetal electronic monitor is applied. In these cases there is confusion as to whether, in the presence of abnormal findings, the labor adds to the damage. Should a cesarean be performed immediately or should a trial of labor ensue? These are questions that cannot answered, but such a finding points to CNS difficulties that predate labor.

Intrapartal Damage and Early Neonatal Function

In general, it is correct to expect that if the fetus was damaged intrapartially, the early neonatal period should be abnormal. Recent stress to the fetus of sufficient degree to cause brain damage is unlikely to leave the neonate with no other signs of abnormality.[1] The converse of that statement is also true. If during the neonatal period observed function is normal, any functional CNS deficits that later are manifested more likely than not did not occur in the intrapartum period.

Using a different model, if the fetal brain is damaged during the antepartum period, it may appear either normal or abnormal during the neonatal period. This depends on how well the fetus recovered from the in utero injury. If the injury took place antepartum, it may not be until much later in infancy until the clinical disability can be identified. Neonatal status and function often do not reflect preexisting clinical pathology.

Relationship of Labor to Cerebral Palsy, Epilepsy, and Mental Retardation

Cerebral Palsy

Cerebral palsy is a nonprogressive motor disorder. In general, the infant with cerebral palsy is not mentally retarded. Cerebral palsy may be associated with an intrapartal event, but is usually not caused by them.[8]

Estimates of the frequency of association between cerebral palsy and perinatal hypoxia vary from 25% to 51%. About one half of the known causes of cerebral palsy occur following nonlabor events. The majority of children who later show cerebral palsy had normal Apgar scores. A depressed Apgar score at 1 minute, but greater than 6 at 5 minutes, is associated with no greater risk for cerebral palsy than a child with normal Apgar scores at 1 and 5 minutes.[10]

Misuse of the Apgar score occurs frequently. The score was never intended to predict brain damage. In a population of infants, a depressed Apgar score has statistical significance. For the individual neonate, the Apgar score is a poor predictor of development. The Apgar score should give direction for fetal treatment to the clinician, but it is not accurate for predicting neurologic function, and a low Apgar score alone is not useful in establishing cause of CNS dysfunction.

Epilepsy and Mental Retardation: Two Different Conditions Less Related to Intrapartal Risk

Epilepsy, an illness unrelated with other neuropathology, such as cerebral palsy, is rarely associated with the birth process. The majority of the causes of epilepsy are unknown.[11] However, that is not the case with the severely damaged infant, who also has convulsions in association with motor pathology; the latter is a diagnosis of cerebral palsy.

Mental retardation, defined as a purely cognitive deficit unassociated with epilepsy or cerebral palsy, is identified as being associated with intrapartal risk in less than 10% of the cases. More often, this pure defect reflects genetic or biochemical events that are not changed by intrapartal manipulations. An infant may have the same mental retardation cognitive effect in association with motor defects and convulsions.

Summary

1. Pathologic findings associated with brain damage
   A. Subdural hematoma

    1. Often associated with trauma

    2. Should rarely occur during intrapartal care

  B. Subarachnoid hemorrhage

    1. Occurs more frequently in the low-birthweight fetus (three times more often than term fetus)

    2. May be related to trauma or hypoxia

    3. May lead to brain damage

  C. Intracerebral hemorrhage

    1. Occurs most frequently in the low-birthweight fetus during neonatal period

    2. Associated with hypoxia and prematurity

    3. May lead to brain damage

  D. Cerebral edema

    1. Seen more commonly in the term infant in the intrapartum period following stress

    2. May lead to brain damage

2. Brain damage syndromes linked with intrapartal care

  A. Cerebral palsy

    1. 50% associated with perinatal risks

    2. 50% associated with low-birthweight fetuses

    3. Significant overlap between categories 1 and 2

    4. Significant percentage follow normal gestation, labor without fetal risk, and have normal Apgar scores

  B. Epilepsy as a pure disease is rarely associated with perinatal or intrapartal events

  C. Mental retardation as a pure disease is rarely associated with perinatal or intrapartal events

3. Brain damage

  A. May be present in some fetuses before labor onset

  B. May be influenced by labor

  C. May occur during the neonatal period in association with prematurity

4. Apgar scores

  A. Do not correlate well with cerebral palsy

  B. Relate to intrapartal fetal distress

References

1. Freeman J. Prenatal and Perinatal Factors Associated with Brain Disorder. Bethesda, MD, National Institutes of Health, publication 85-1149, April, 1985.

2. Rosen MG, Hobel CJ. Prenatal and perinatal factors associated with brain disorders. Obstet Gynecol 1986;68:416–421.

3. Pape KE, Wigglesworth SS. Hemorrhage, Ischemia and the Perinatal Brain. London, Heinemann, 1979.

4. Rosen MG, Bilenker RM, Thompson K. An assessment of developmental time periods and risk for brain damage in fetus and infant. J Reprod Med 1986;31:297–303.

5. Banker BQ, Laffoche JC. Periventricular leukoencephalomalacia of infancy. A form of anoxic encephalopathy. Arch Neurol 1962;7:386–410.

6. Pape KE, Armstrong DL, Fitzhardinge PM. Central nervous system pathology associated with mask ventilation in the very low birthweight infant: A new etiology of intracerebral hemorrhages. Pediatrics 1976;58:473–483.

7. Westgmn M, Paul R. Delivery of the low birth weight infant by cesarean section. Clin Obstet Gynecol 1985;28:752–762.

8. Kiely M, Labin RA, Kiely JL. The descriptive epidemiology of cerebral palsy. Public Health Rev 1984;12:79–101.

9. Hagberg G, Hagberg B, Chow I. The changing panorama of cerebral palsy in Sweden, 1954–1970. III. The importance of foetal deprivation of supply. Acta Paediatr Scand 1976;65:403–408.

10. Nelson KB, Enenberg JH. Apgar scores as predictors of cerebral palsy. Pediatrics 1981;68:36–44.

11. Hauser WA, Kuriand LT. Epidemiology of epilepsy in Rochester, Minn, 1935–1986. Epilepsia 1975;16:1–66.

Chapter 3

Preadmission and Admission Responsibilities: A Guide to Care in Labor

Overview

Confusion in the use of terms such as *perinatal* and *neonatal asphyxia, anoxia, hypoxia,* and their relationships to the etiology of brain damage have been described. Terminology for labor and the definitions of labor diagnoses are used in this textbook as a dictionary of descriptive terms for patient care. If there are standardized clinical definitions to use when abnormal clinical courses have been encountered, it is easier to decide on an appropriate course of action in the intrapartum period. When you exceed expected normal parameters, you act. Actions should follow objective information, not just a subjective feeling, for example, "the head won't fit." True cephalopelvic disproportion, though present, can only be speculated on, even after the neonate has been delivered. In contrast, failure of the vertex to descend after full cervical dilatation is definable in terms of time.

In this text, Friedman's labor definitions are used as they are derived from his original calculations performed at Presbyterian Hospital and Columbia University College of Physicians and Surgeons in New York.[1] In more recent studies of women during labor performed at Cleveland Metropolitan General Hospital by Dr. David Peisner together with the original author of this treatise, Dr. Mort Rosen, comparisons with Friedman's original observations were remarkably consistent.[2] In a few instances, such as in the latent phase of labor, practical clinical modifications are introduced. However, throughout this text the Friedman criteria are used as guidelines for documenting what is taking place in labor. Clinical intervention, made in association with labor diagnosis, involves the use of good judgment performed at the bedside by the clinician. Too often the Friedman guidelines have been used as a reason for terminating labor because the patient does not conform to the usual lengths of latent, active, or second stages of labor.[3] Falling outside of a numerical range alone does not document significant risk for brain injury and does not, in and of itself, warrant an automatic clinical intervention.

Objectives

At the conclusion of this chapter, the clinician should understand and be able to describe the following:

1. Labor terminology and graphing of the progress of labor
2. Appropriate general conduct of personnel in the labor and delivery room
   a. Obligations of the physician
   b. Use of monitoring
   c. Charting and documentation of clinical events

Chart Notes

Labor takes place over a period of many hours, during which the clinician is responsible for the patient's health care. Comprehensive chart notes during the course of labor enable the physician to review his or her earlier thoughts intelligently. It helps the clinician plan for and anticipate the progress of labor and recall what took place earlier. Memory of events considered important at some point earlier in labor may not be as clear in the middle of the night. Years later, when the record might be reviewed, a logical process for patient care can be more easily validated. In summary, complete chart notes both facilitate and document the process of decision making. Chart notes, with date and time of day, also document your attendance in the labor room, which is an important documentation for many reasons.

Labor Graphs

The labor graph should be constructed while labor is in progress (Fig. 3.1). The graph presents a visual picture of labor, which helps the clinician understand patient progress and quickly determine the stage of labor. The labor graph allows obstetrical personnel to intervene promptly, if necessary. It replaces subjective terms such as *good labor* or *poor progress* with an objective slope of cervical dilatation. A *good labor* in the active phase should have a nearly vertical slope of dilatation. The labor graph also allows the viewer to conceptualize the relationship between cervical dilatation and vertex descent. Descent and vertex engagement often occur late in labor. Many clinicians assume that active-phase labor without vertex engagement is unusual, but in fact it is quite common, especially in multiparous women, and is easily documented when graphing becomes routine.

Meaning of Labor Progress Numbers

The numbers defining progress in labor are guidelines and should be used with caution. By themselves, labors varying outside the standard deviations, means,

22

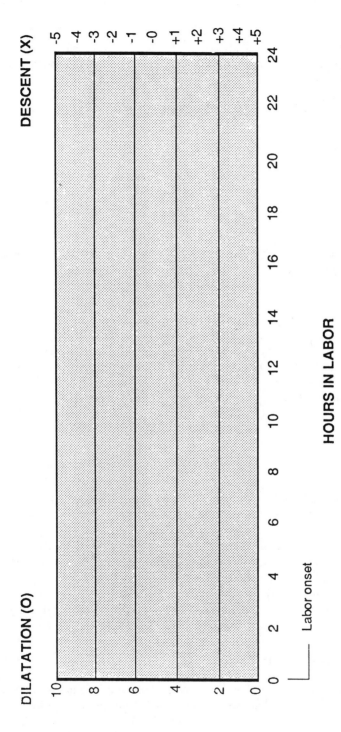

FIGURE 3.1

and medians of large population studies do not indicate clinical complication or any minor risk for neurologic morbidity. For example, a person may be short and differ from the mean height of all people, or be two standard deviations shorter than the average person. Yet, although short, that individual is still a normal and healthy person. One may not infer that because of height the very short person is sick. A labor graph that documents a labor that "falls off" the Friedman curve and does not conform to the usual labor progress expected does not mean that fetal damage has occurred or will occur.

Abnormal numbers in the latent or active phase of labor, such as prolongations, protractions, or arrests, are signals to assess whether interventions are needed. Alerted by the numbers and the visual graph, the obstetrician understands that the patient's labor is not proceeding in the typical way and the labor warrants attention. Objective information about the course of labor can alert the physician to atypical progress, and the physician can then attempt to decipher the cause and intervene in a timely fashion. Since clinical care is improved by intervention at the correct time, this information then can be directly linked to an improved quality of care. Deviations from standard graphical labor patterns have been used by some clinicians as a reason to terminate labor abruptly. However, when protractions or arrests are identified, the judgment of the physician should involve a consideration of various treatments that might affect normal vaginal delivery. It is only after such treatment choices have been appropriately considered and rejected or found unsuccessful that terminating labor by cesarean delivery is acceptable.

General Conduct in the Labor and Delivery Room

Education for Childbirth and Support During Labor

It has been established that a prepared mother manages the birthing experience more easily than an unprepared mother.[4] Labor and delivery support persons have historically been husbands. Today there is no reason why a properly motivated alternative support person (friend, family member, or professional assistant) cannot assist the laboring mother. There is adequate information suggesting that labors are more easily managed, patients enjoy the experience more, and perhaps even the incidence of abnormal labor may be lowered in a more friendly birthing environment. However, the key word is *support*. Individuals who wish to attend labor and delivery because they are merely curious or wish to be entertained may cause more distraction than help.

Childbirth education is almost universally available. It is important that the information being taught is consistent with the procedures to which the patient will be exposed. There are times when physicians' procedures are not the same as those being taught in prenatal courses. It is the obligation of the medical staff (nurses, midwives, and physicians) to attempt to present a nonconfusing and consistent educational program. Ingrained in this must be physician flexibility and patient choice.

It cannot be overemphasized that the full spectrum of labor information should be taught. An idealized version of the best of all outcomes may hinder a patient's adaptation if idealized labor does not take place. Some women may tolerate labor with little medication or anesthesia; some will not. The patient, suddenly confused by what, to her, is unexpected pain, may adapt to the labor poorly. Patient frustration, fear, and fatigue may influence management and can result in early termination of labor unnecessarily. The prepared mother, educated to the full spectrum of potential labor events, including the pain of contractions, is more easily supported during labor. It is important for the physician to be fully aware of what is being taught in the childbirth education courses his or her patient attends.

EXAMPLE OF A POTENTIAL FOR CONFUSION IN TYPE OF LABOR ROOM SUPPORT

Two patients were overheard in the same physician's waiting room discussing their breathing exercises for labor. One patient described a series of five patterns she was being taught. The second was being taught a single breathing exercise for all of labor.

Comment

During labor, support for the patient after such varied educational programs will be difficult, since specific information taught to any individual patient is unknown to the support personnel.

Patient Treatment Routines

Flexibility in treatment implies that no single pattern of care will apply to all patients.

EXAMPLE OF PATTERNED MEDICATION USE

Some physicians medicate all mothers using a fixed routine beginning at entry into the labor room, and supplemented every several hours thereafter in order to provide analgesia during labor.

Comment

This is a clinical care pattern best relegated to history. Judgment suggests that for different mothers in different labors, different analgesic regimens might be needed. Patient care should be individualized.

EXAMPLE OF INDIVIDUALIZED CARE

At 4 cm of cervical dilation, a mother may request medication. In the low-risk healthy patient, this allows the clinician wide variability of choice. Patient choice should predominate.

Comment

The kind of pain relief used will be dictated by the labor progress the clinician perceives is taking place and by the patient's needs and desires. The mother with a high vertex may be given 50 mg of meperidine intravenously to assist in relaxation between contractions. The mother with a well-engaged vertex may be offered an epidural block to remove the discomfort of contractions. A third mother may be tolerating the latent phase well and need no analgesic medication at this time.

In uncomplicated cases, the average cervical dilatation for a patient to be ready to be admitted to the labor and delivery room is approximately 4 cm. Admitting patients too early in labor should generally be avoided. In uncomplicated cases, early labor may be better tolerated at home and less medication may be required.

Physician Presence During Labor and Delivery

Each physician will have different patterns for patient attention and for being present during the stages of labor. This will depend on the hospital environment, the support staff, and the patient. Whether the physician is present or not, responsibility for the patient remains with her physician. That "contract" was established with the first antepartum visit, and the resulting responsibility continues until after the pregnancy is safely terminated and the patient has fully recovered, or until that responsibility is transferred to and accepted by another physician.

If Risk Is Present During Labor

In uncomplicated cases, the clinician should be readily available for consultation if an unexpected risk develops. In the presence of significant risk to the mother or fetus, the clinician should be physically present in order to perform a personal evaluation. If the physician cannot or chooses not to be present, a competent alternate care provider must be chosen.

EXAMPLE OF ACUTE FETAL RISK AND PHYSICIAN PRESENCE

Telephone notification is received from the labor admitting nurse that there is a fetal heart pattern indicative of repetitive variable decelerations in a patient who is in early labor.

Comment

The obstetrician's personal presence is required to review the clinical situation until it is stabilized. If the physician chooses to have the situation evaluated by another responsible person while he/she is not physically present, that is a decision that should be most carefully made. As a responsible clinician, it is understood that while patient evaluation may be transferred, the responsibility for patient care (the results of the evaluation and subsequent decision) is not transferable. If the authority for making clinical decisions is transferred and inappropriate decisions are made, the responsibility remains with the patient's obstetrician*.

EXAMPLE OF CHRONIC FETAL RISK AND PHYSICIAN PRESENCE

The patient arrived in the labor screening area with ruptured membranes. Pea soup meconium-stained amniotic fluid was described to the obstetrician by the examining nurse.

Comment

While the actual fetal risk for the release of that meconium may have taken place hours or days earlier, the condition should be evaluated at the bedside until a decision as to the severity of the problem is reached and a judgment concerning patient care is made.

Can the obstetrician stay in an office in a building nearby, or an office connected to the hospital, or on the floor below the labor unit as the labor continues? That is a clinical judgment only the obstetrician can make after evaluating an individual patient. If the clinician has doubts, obviously the answer is to stay with the patient. The attending physician should write a timed and dated chart note describing clinical findings and impressions at the time of evaluating the patient as well as specific plans for intervention if appropriate.

If Labor Is Normal

The clinician will rarely stay at the bedside continuously through labor. Some people may argue that the physician should always be present, but the facts speak for themselves. It is not practical for a physician to remain at the patient's side throughout labor. The labor room environment and support system for patient care must be factors in the physician's decision to be present or not.

In the presence of a normal uncomplicated labor, "physician presence" has more latitude. Early in the latent phase of the labor of a vertex fetal presentation, greater choice exists. In contrast, with a breech presentation the situation should be managed differently. Although stated facetiously, perhaps one of the major improve-

---

*While the care is described as being given by the individual physician, it is understood that in group practices the responsibility remains within the group, although at any one time it is assumed by an individual physician.

ments in obstetrical patient care was introducing adequate lounge and sleeping facilities so that obstetrician can be comfortable in the labor room environment.

Today, the number of group practices continues to grow. In large groups physicians are sometimes assigned to labor rooms on a fulltime basis. This constant attention is more "time" expensive, but good quality care can be more easily maintained. This, of course, is impractical except in groups with a large number of obstetrical personnel.

Because the physician has so frequently chosen, or has been unable to stay at, the bedside, nurses, midwives, and other labor partners have filled this void. There is little doubt that this personalized support relieves anxiety, makes the labor more tolerable, and may shorten the labor. Sharing bedside support and care with appropriate professional staff is not only appropriate, it can improve patient care.

Responsibility for Patient Care

It may be thought by some that the authority and responsibility for the outcome of bedside care for the patient can be transferred to other persons, such as nurses or resident physicians. In the event of a problem, it is the attending obstetrician's responsibility, whether in the labor room, in the building next door, or at home. Once again, responsibility is not transferrable.

Chart Documentation: Record Keeping

Hospital chart review makes clear that deficiencies in documentation are common. When charts are reviewed for hospital quality assurance programs, educational case discussions, research purposes, or courtroom appearances, all too often they contain less than adequate physician's notes. In fact, far more extensive effort, care, and attention usually is provided by physicians than is recorded in the medical chart. Nurses have generally been trained to "chart" more frequently and completely than physicians, but the changing legal environment requires physicians to chart more comprehensively than has been common in the past. Notes, findings, and thoughts are important and should be expressed in writing. As mentioned earlier, notes should be complete—dated and timed—and written soon after the evaluation or intervention is performed.

Admission to Labor and Delivery: A First Evaluation

On admission to the labor room, a comprehensive evaluation should be performed. This assessment should include a general history and physical evaluation written in the hospital chart. Statements should be made about the estimated size of the fetus, its position, the maternal phase of labor, and the quality and timing of contractions. If there are deviations from the usual and expected findings, these should be noted.

Table 3.1   Notes for Admission*

1. Date and time of writing note
2. Patient description of labor history
3. Significant historical data
4. General physical examination
5. Obstetrical examination
6. Evaluation of labor and prognosis

*Complete this note shortly after the examination.

Patient Plan Following the Admission Note (Table 3.1)

It is helpful to estimate what is anticipated in the course of labor. Is a normal course of labor expected? If different management than typical is anticipated, what is the basis for such management? Explicitly stating expectations will not only improve this predictive process with experience, but also the written record is established as a base for later patient care.

EXAMPLE OF COMPLETION OF ADMISSION NOTE BY THE RESPONSIBLE PHYSICIAN

Someone else has already examined the patient and an admission note has been written for you by a resident or nurse. This note may be your first chart entry.

4/20/96, 0100: The patient states her contractions began 1900 hours on 4/19. The abdominal examination confirms a vertex presentation with the back in the left side and vertex dipping into the pelvis. The estimated fetal weight is 7 lb. On vaginal examination the vertex is at station 2. The membranes are intact; the cervix is 3 cm dilated and 90% effaced. The patient is probably in the latent phase of labor. (Note: You must observe cervical dilatation to confirm labor.) I anticipate no problems. The patient has requested that no monitoring be performed unless necessary. The use of monitoring has been discussed during office visits, and the patient's request is accepted.

Comment

In this example, the clinician's note did not include the patient's past history or physical examination. In this case, it was inferred that the information had already been obtained by others and read by the patient's responsible physician. It would be appropriate to state, "Admitting information reviewed and agreed with."

If no earlier evaluation has taken place, important data should be obtained; a short note would include relevant historical information, vital signs, and pertinent physical findings. Most accreditation agencies require a complete history, including a social history and a physical examination. This base history can be appropriately satisfied with a prenatal history form and a recent update.

The decision against electronic monitoring infers an adequate auscultation support system. In the normal patient, the use of electronic monitoring is a clinical judgment and need not be arbitrarily performed. There must, as noted, be adequate support to provide auscultation approximately every 30 minutes during latent-phase labor, and every 15 minutes during active-phase. The auscultated information should be charted.

Progress Notes

As labor progresses, additional written observations are helpful. Should these notes be written hourly? Probably not. An entry should be made whenever any significant observation or any intervention occurs. Frequency of notation is determined by patient progress and the presence of normal or problem situations. Review the earlier notes. It is always helpful to review earlier thoughts.

Some clinician's have suggested that hourly vaginal examinations should be the rule. In latent labor this is clearly not necessary. In active labor, timing of examination should be determined individually based on labor progress and the patient's individual risk factors.

EXAMPLE OF A PROGRESS NOTE

4/20/96, 1300: At 0900 the patient was 8 cm dilated with vertex at –3 station. Since that time this patient has made no progress. An arrest of cervical dilation and descent of the vertex in the active phase is present. On clinical examination, the patient's pelvis appears adequate for this fetus. Contractions are occurring every 4 minutes and are of poor quality. Oxytocin will be used to overcome this arrest of labor. Fetal monitoring has revealed no signs of non-reassuring fetal status.

Comment

Some practitioners might not have allowed the arrest to continue beyond 2 hours before the original intervention (oxytocin). Some might have medicated the patient. Others would have ended the oxytocin augmentation after 1 hour if progress did not take place. The final decision in this case was to perform a cesarean. Later in time, by reading the clinical notes, a quality assessment committee or an attorney would know the condition of the fetus during the arrest and why the decision was made. During the hours of patient care, the presence of the physicians' notes enables the clinician to review the reasoning process. Two or 3 years after the birth, in the absence of complete notes, it will not be possible to reconstruct the process, and, even if attempted, it may not be believed without a written record.

There is no specific time to end a trial of labor. In the presence of a normal pregnancy, lack of non-reassuring fetal status by fetal monitoring, and absent meconium during labor, most clinicians would not criticize this patient's care. In the presence of other risks, the clinician may have ended labor earlier. Electronic monitoring was appropriate as there was an "other than usual" labor pattern (an indication for monitoring) and because oxytocin was used (an indication for monitoring).

Electronic Fetal Monitoring

Ensuring the availability of monitoring at the hospital where labor is planned, and a discussion of its use and its limitations, should have taken place during the antenatal period. Although rarely recorded in charts, it is helpful to have both antenatal and intrapartal notes documenting a discussion as to whether monitoring should be used.

The benefits of electronic fetal monitoring (EFM) continue to be controversial. In the low-risk patient, in the absence of intrapartal problems and the presence of adequate support persons for auscultation (listening each 30 minutes during latent phase, each 5 minutes during active phase), there is no evidence that the use of EFM reduces risk or improves long-term outcome. Its use, however, is associated with an increase in cesarean delivery rate. There may also be a slight decrease in the evidence of neonatal seizures. There has been no demonstration of a reduction in the incidence of cerebral palsy.

EXAMPLE OF DOCUMENTATION OF FETAL MONITORING REQUEST
(INTRAPARTUM NOTE)

Earlier during pregnancy, Mrs. Smith and I discussed the use of fetal monitoring. We discussed this again this evening in her labor room with her husband. They understand the reasons for monitoring use, including its potential value in some unpredictable labor problems such as occlusion of the umbilical cord. They prefer no use of electronic monitoring.

Comment

The antenatal record should document the discussions. Later, recall by the patient of monitoring discussions occurring only during a period of tension in the labor room may be quite different.

Many hospitals have rules requiring electronic monitoring of all patients. Other hospitals allow flexibility in the absence of fetal risk. There are arguments to support each philosophy. There has been little change in knowledge about monitoring since the publication entitled *Antenatal Diagnosis: Intrapartum Fetal Distress* by the National Institutes of Health in 1979.[5] Therefore, choice for monitoring use is still appropriate. Until the time comes when monitoring may take place so easily that it is neither cumbersome not burdensome to patients and staff, and the use of the information is so clear that error in use of monitoring is lessened, it is preferable to offer a choice to the low-risk patient in uncomplicated labor.

The Hospital

Early in pregnancy the patient should be made aware of the hospital's capabilities for backup support. If a hospital exists in an environment where other hospitals are not accessible, patient choice of a hospital to labor in is obviously limited. In contrast, if several hospitals exist near enough to permit patient choice, and different levels of medical support are present at the adjacent hospitals, information should be given to the patient in order to assist her in making an informed choice.

Patient concerns may include the availability of in-hospital anesthesiologists, emergency operating-room facilities, and neonatal support systems, as well as the availability of rooming-in, breastfeeding support, and other educational support systems. This information should be part of the childbirth education program. An opportunity to visit the labor and delivery room environment and meet the nursing staff should be part of this education program.

Patient Sensitivity and Patient Information

Although awareness of patient sensitivity is basic to clinical care, it cannot be overemphasized that respect for privacy, personal rights, and free exchange of information is expected. No longer is the physician allowed to introduce clinical care and expect treatment to be accepted without explanation. It is easier to exchange information before carrying out intervention rather than afterwards, especially if a complication has occurred.

It is rare for a patient to absolutely demand an alternate to the medical care recommended by her physician. As the physician, you are not giving up your right to provide medical care or to utilize your professional judgment by reviewing and discussing the problem with the patient. To the contrary, sharing information is part of the process of appropriate medical care. However, no matter how the treatment is explained, the responsibility for the outcome will be the physician's. If the patient absolutely refuses to accept a medical recommendation, the risks of such refusal should be clearly explained and documented in the medical record.

Privacy and personal feelings in the labor room environment must be protected. Statements such as "Please," "Thank you," "May I come in?" and "May I examine you?" (closing the door when you do), may be lost in a busy labor and delivery suite. Yet, long after the birth has occurred, many patients raise questions totally unexpected by the physician, but extremely important to the mother, indicating that these are extremely critical aspects of what a patient perceives as caring, high-quality care.

EXAMPLE OF PATIENT CHOICE IN A BREECH PRESENTATION

At term, a P3 G2 mother in latent labor with the cervix 4 cm dilated and at –2 station is informed that the fetus is in a frank breech presentation. A vertex presentation had been presumed during the antepartum period.

Comment

A discussion of choice for vaginal or cesarean birth should be initiated. In the situation where there is disagreement among physicians as to how the breech should be delivered, the patient should be informed of the alternatives in treatment philosophies. This is a classic situation in which patient choice often resolves the question, but the physician often influences the outcome by the manner in which the information is presented. It is important that risks and benefits of appropriate options be presented to the patient. It is also important to inform the patient of your recommendation and the basis for it.

Because of their concern about high cesarean birthrates, some physicians wisely discuss potential problem situations at the onset of patient care. Situations such as abnormal labor progress, fetal distress, and previous cesareans are often reviewed prior to labor. Patient understanding of information presented in a non–tension-filled environment (antepartum) makes decision regarding patient care during labor much easier.

EXAMPLE OF BIASING A PATIENT'S CHOICE

Mrs. Kelly is given all the information about the baby's breech position and the risks to the baby associated with a vaginal breech delivery.

Comment

That is no choice. Mrs. Kelly will respond, "I want a cesarean to protect my child." The patient decision, biased by the manner in which the physician introduced the information, will usually be to perform the cesarean. Yet, the patient must know the potential risks and benefits involved in each option. It is not easy to fully discuss and explain the probability of a complication that is possible but uncommon, and this is well understood by all experienced clinicians.

EXAMPLE OF BIASING A PATIENT'S CHOICE

Mrs. Kelly is given the pertinent information about the baby's breech position and the risks to both the mother, and fetus associated with both vaginal and cesarean delivery. In addition, she is also told that it is believed this baby will do as well when born by the vaginal birth route as by any alternative intervention.

Comment

This presents a different choice, but this too is not yet free from physician bias. This example more often will result in a vaginal delivery. The first example, with the inclusion of all potential specific fetal risks and little apparent alternatives to the cesarean, perhaps explains why so many breech presentations are delivered abdominally.

There must be a middle route between these two examples of presenting the risks without exaggeration and in a balanced manner. When there is no absolute answer, it is a patient choice situation. The breech presentation is often such an example.

EXAMPLE OF A SITUATION WHERE THERE SHOULD BE NO PATIENT CHOICE

A P1 G2 mother, at term, presents in labor actively bleeding bright-red blood. About 600 ml of blood have been estimated to have been lost since the onset of contractions. Electronic fetal monitoring reveals repeated late decelerations following each contraction.

Comment

The patient is quickly informed of the need for a rapid evaluation to find the etiology of the hemorrhage. This situation still requires an information exchange, but, in contrast to the breech presentation, appropriate patient choice is severely limited. All necessary steps should be instituted to provide rapid resolution of the problem. The patient should not debate the issue, nor should she take away the physician's rights in emergency decisions. Exchange of the information in this case takes place in a different manner.

Following situations such as the previous example, when decisions have been made rapidly, often in the midst of a medical crisis, patient emotional turmoil often develops. Follow-up discussions during the immediate postcrisis or postpartum period should take place. Lack of post–cesarean-delivery discussion frequently results in the patient requesting a repeat cesarean when given a choice for a trial of labor in a subsequent pregnancy. The fear engendered by the first (failed) labor and surgery, or fetal concerns not understood or resolved, may lead to fear for recurrence. In a subsequent pregnancy, why should she choose labor having this concern when the elective cesarean seems so simple?

Labor and Delivery Room Environment

The labor room environment can be either emotionally supportive or disturbing. Sounds from adjacent laboring patients can be frightening. Physicians' conversations about labor-related issues (when not explained), or casual discussions about other patients or nonlabor events may be perceived by the laboring mother in a very different frame of reference than by the speakers. Laughing over jokes, or even odors from foods cooked in a nearby microwave oven, can be upsetting to the individual patient or her family.

EXAMPLE OF INFORMATION REQUESTED LONG AFTER LABOR

One year following a cesarean delivery because of hypertensive encephalopathy, a mother requested an opportunity to return to the labor and recovery rooms. This came as a surprise to the physician, who began to elucidate more information relating to this request.

Comment

On further questioning, the physician learned that the patient had no recollection of the 48-hour period during which she had been critically ill. One year later, she still had recurring nightmares about what might have taken place during the time she was mentally obtunded. She wished to see the rooms and people she could not remember.

EXAMPLE OF MISUNDERSTANDING A HALLWAY DISCUSSION

A discussion of the fetal distress that was occurring in patient A's labor took place outside the doorway of patient B's room. Patient B heard the conversation and concluded that this "fetal distress" referred to her son.

Comment

Despite a normal labor and delivery, the mother raised her child with the internalized fears that he was different and needed more help and understanding because he had incurred fetal distress. Her son was always referred to as her "sick child." No one realized that she had heard the adjacent patient's problems being discussed by the staff. The obstetrician learned of her fears years later during a casual conversation taking place at an annual checkup. Review of her labor records confirmed that there had been no fetal distress.

Fetal Distress and Emergency Cesarean

In contrast to an imagined problem, if a problem such as "fetal distress" should occur, the meaning of this term should be discussed with the patient again after the completion of labor. In the postoperative period, to the patient the term *fetal distress* implies risk and trauma. The actions taken during labor to evaluate and treat a problem often shift control of labor from the patient to medical personnel. The patient is told to turn from one side to the other. Suddenly, an oxygen mask is placed over her nose and mouth. In the extreme case, the abdomen is rapidly shaved, a Foley catheter is inserted, and she is rolled into a new room—the operating room. Among new persons, often without her husband, the patient is rapidly placed under anesthesia. It is little wonder that many patients are physically and psychologically traumatized by labor events and are determined not to undergo labor again.

It should be pointed out that a fetal heart-rate recording described as non-reassuring does not necessarily result in a later development abnormality. In fact, in the vast majority of such cases there are no subsequent developmental abnormalities. It is an indication that a period of increased observation is needed to avoid increasing fetal risk. Fetal distress or non-reassuring fetal status, (more properly) may mean fetal risk; it rarely means fetal damage. Fetal distress concerning a patient should not be discussed where a second patient may overhear. In labors when the diagnosis of fetal distress leads to surgery, the parents need a complete discussion of the events that took place and, when possible, need to be reassured that the infant's future is optimistic. This should take place on several occasions during the postpartum period and be repeated at the 6-week visit. Lack of information creates more fear than do explained problems.

Summary

1. The Friedman labor definitions are used throughout this text.

2. Definitions are guides to interventions and not rules that must be adhered to.

3. Active plotting of labor graphs allows for improved clinical evaluation and education of all personnel.

4. The conduct of all labor room personnel and the physical and emotional support systems for patients during labor are integral parts of patient care.

5. In the presence of fetal risk, or until the fetal risk is evaluated, the obstetrician should be with the patient.

6. Electronic fetal monitoring is appropriate with at-risk patients and is optional for normal patients.

7. Admission and progress notes should be written by the clinician because they are helpful during patient care and invaluable for later review.

8. Sensitivity to patient needs and a supportive labor room environment are also a physician's responsibility.

References

1. Friedman EA. Labor: Clinical Evaluation and Management, ed 2. New York, Appleton-Century-Crofts, 1978.

2. Peisner DB, Rosen MG. The latent phase of labor in normal patients: A reassessment. Obstet Gynecol 1985;66:644–648.

3. Peisner DB, Rosen MG. Transition from latent to active labor. Obstet Gynecol 1986;68:448–500.

4. Sosa R, Kennell J, Klaus M, Robertson S, Urrutia J. The effect of a supportive companion on perinatal problems, length of labor, and mother-infant interaction. N Engl J Med 1980;303:597–600.

5. Antenatal Diagnosis: Intrapartum Fetal Distress. Bethesda, MD, National Institutes of Child Health and Human Development, publication 79-1973, 1979.

Chapter 4

The Clinical Examination

Overview

The clinical examination includes the patient's general history and physical examination, performed for all patients upon admission to the hospital, as well as the obstetrical examination. Because the laboring patient has usually been seen and examined completely during the previous year, the contents of the general history and physical examination may be condensed, introducing only pertinent or new information. In contrast, the obstetrical examination must not be neglected or simplified too often occurs. A complete obstetrical examination, including an abdominal examination and a repeat clinical pelvimetry if necessary, should be performed in every patient who is in or suspected of being in labor.

Objectives

At this conclusion of this chapter, the clinician should recognize the need for the following:

1. Documentation of important historical information and general physical findings of patients in labor that may impact on the labor, delivery, or postpartum course

2. A complete obstetrical examination to evaluate the patient and to develop a plan for the completion of labor, including

   a. Abdominal examination

   b. Vaginal examination

   c. Clinical pelvimetry

3. Ultrasonography as a supportive laboratory test for the clinical examination

4. The limitations of x-ray pelvimetry

General History and Physical Examination

In the impersonal world of technologic medicine, the obstetrician has a unique opportunity to establish a close personal relationship with the patient. This is initiated at the first prenatal visit, and it grows with each subsequent prenatal visit. The culmination of this relationship is the sensitive and often demanding association between the patient, her family, and the obstetrician during labor. Overemphasis on technology may result in destruction of this sensitive relationship if improperly used. Today it is a unique situation to be able to examine a patient in early labor without the presence of an already in-place monitoring system covering her abdomen. It is not unusual to have the pelvic examination followed by abdominal ultrasonography without complete patient evaluation ever taking place. Although the patient in labor has already undergone a thorough history and physical examination, the process must be respected. A review of the patient's interval history should take place, that recent illness, medications, and diet. Unusual allergies or illness should then be reconfirmed and drug use recorded in the chart note. A general physical examination, including vital signs, heart and lung evaluations, mental acuity, presence of drugs, and neurologic reflexes should take place. If the physical examination is normal, this should be noted, as well as all positive findings.

Obstetrical Evaluation

Observation

Observe the patient and look at her abdomen. By the time many clinicians see their patients in labor, the patients' abdomens are covered with various external belts. It is quite helpful to look at the maternal abdomen and begin to determine the following:

1. Fetal size: Although it may be just an estimate, it can be an early warning of a large or small fetus.
2. Fetal lie: Long before ultrasonography is used, an oblique or transverse lie can be suspected by looking at the abdomen. An unusual presentation can be confirmed with ultrasonography after the physical examination is completed.
3. Fetal position: Before the manual abdominal examination is performed, there should be an attempt to visualize on which side the fetal back lies. When medical students or residents are asked to look at the maternal abdomen of a seventh or eighth month patient and point to the side the fetal back is on, they inevitably choose the round side rather than the correct side. The back, when it can be seen in late pregnancy, is the straight side of the maternal abdomen; the arms and legs produce the round convexity.

EXAMPLE OF AN ABDOMINAL EXAMINATION COMPLIMENTING THE VAGINAL EXAMINATION

A primigravid woman at 38 weeks of gestation was in the active phase of labor, 6 cm dilated with vertex at –3 station. Abdominal observation noted the straight side was on the left and the round side on the right (therefore, the back was on the left side.) Following vaginal examination, the examiner was uncertain if the vertex was right occiput anterior (ROA) or left occiput posterior (LOP), as the head was not flexed and the fontanels could not be easily felt.

Comment

The answer was straightforward. Knowing that the fetal back was on the left side following the clinical examination would have eliminated the confusion. In vertex presentation, the back and the occiput are on the same side. This finding would also allow the clinician to anticipate a longer time to delivery, as it takes more time for the occiput posterior fetus to rotate and descend.

Similarly, "looking" while a patient is bearing down during the second stage of labor is also helpful.

EXAMPLE OF VISUALIZING VAGINAL DILATION DURING STAGE OF LABOR

A G3 P2 mother with a fully dilated cervix and vertex at +2 station was voluntarily pushing with each contraction. At the height of each pushing effort, everyone was anticipating caput. It was obvious that the labia were separating during her expulsive efforts. However, there was no caput visible. In this circumstance, even without a vaginal digital examination, using your "observation," you would know a wider diameter of the fetal vertex is presenting. Thus, either a larger vertex or an occiput transverse or posterior is present. The larger diameters of the presenting vertex in these situations distend the labia before the caput is visible. The birth will take longer until descent, either with or without rotation, takes place and before crowning is seen.

Palpate the Abdomen: The Four Maneuvers of Leopold

The abdominal examination should be performed before the vaginal examination. If not, it may be neglected. Many physicians have incorrectly estimated the vertex position or have even missed the presenting part because of failure to pursue a complete clinical examination. The abdominal examination is best performed by utilizing the four maneuvers of Leopold described below:

1. Palpate the fundus and estimate its height, or preferably, measure it with a tape measure. The height of the fundus determined by the examiner's

hands is a good estimator of fetal size. This is always modified by whether or not membranes are ruptured, the patient's size, or the fetal lie. The examination is least accurate in the presence of unusual fetal positions, or at the extremes of fetal weight.

If there is uncertainty as to whether the fetal part in the fundus is the breech, continue gently holding the fundus with one or both hands for several moments. Holding on to the breech is often associated with kicking or palpable movements of the fetal extremities that are not felt with the vertex. Fetal heart deceleration associated with pressure or squeezing on the vertex has not been as helpful. In many labor rooms the ultrasound machine can and should be used as needed. However, the clinical examination still has its place.

2. The second movement of Leopold is facilitated by the impression of the fetal lie from earlier observations and palpation's. While still facing the maternal head, run both hands along the sides of the uterus. Palpation of the back is facilitated by earlier impressions of visualizing the straight side and the often moving extremities on the opposite side.

3. Still facing the patient's head, grasp the presenting part and attempt to move it. It may be immovable and well fixed in the pelvis (possibly engaged) or easily movable (probably not engaged). This is an uncomfortable procedure for the patient and may stimulate an urge to void. Be gentle in trying to reach low enough behind the pubic symphysis to complete this maneuver.

4. Turn towards the patient's feet and with both hands moving along the sides of the vertex, note whether the examining hands begin to converge (unengaged if the top of the head is reached) or diverge (possibly engaged). In the uncommon face presentation, the hyperextended head may be palpated on the same side as the back.

5. The above discussion may appear almost insignificant in today's technology-oriented labor room. However, there is no obstetrician who at times has not been uncertain as to fetal vertex position. Use everything that is available, that is, the clinical art of obstetrics.

General Vaginal Examination

This examination is performed with sterile gloves but without additional washing or preparation of the perineum, which has never been documented as increasing sterility of the exam. The vaginal examination is the final step in documenting the fetal position and predicting the progress of the labor. Complete clinical pelvimetry, or clinical measurements of the pelvis, are not usually undertaken during routine labor examinations unless there is a question or concern about the initial clinical pelvimetry performed at the first antenatal visit. During labor the patient is uncomfortable, pelvic muscle relaxation not attainable, and the vertex may be in the way of the clinician's attempt to measure the diagonal conjugate. On the other hand, should the examiner suspect there is a feto-pelvic disproportion at any time during the labor process, a careful, if abbreviated, repeat clinical pelvimetry should be undertaken.

Fundal pressure may allow an estimate of how easily the vertex may descend into the pelvis later. If the vertex descends with fundal pressure and reaches or exceeds the levels of the ischial spines, fetal and pelvic size should not be an anticipated problem. This maneuver is a guide, though, not an absolute answer.

During the later vaginal examinations, an estimate may be made of how much room there is in the pelvis by noting space around the vertex and in the hollow of the sacrum. The examination should be performed while thinking in terms of pelvic capacity, not pelvic measurement. Is the pelvis large enough? Is there room around the head? Does the head descend? If the examination is performed only to measure cervical dilatation and to assess vertex station, then the physician may incorrectly believe, as some have suggested, that clinical examination for pelvic assessment is useless.

Vaginal Examination of the Cervix and Presenting Part

The vaginal examination during labor should also disclose cervical effacement, dilatation, the presenting part and its position, and the relationship between the presenting part and the ischial spines.

Cervical effacement is measured by percentages or gross estimates, and gives important information as to labor length. The length of the cervix varies from patient to patient. For uniformity assume the cervix to be 2 cm in length when uneffaced. By measuring the length of the cervix remaining, a percentage can be applied for the amount of effacement. A 40% or 50% thick cervix foreshadows a longer labor. A cervix almost 100% effaced foreshadows a much shorter labor.

Cervical dilatation is usually estimated based on an arbitrary assignment of 10 cm as complete dilatation. As a result, it is often best to measure the exact dilation up to 5 cm, and then after 5 cm to measure the remaining cervix and subtract that from 10 to estimate the dilatation. The cervix will have a slow rate of dilatation during latent phase, and a more rapid rate in active phase. Also, is the cervix anterior or posterior? If the cervix is well behind or posterior, anticipate a longer time for dilatation.

Vertex position is next evaluated. Think of the position of the fontanels. Identifying their location allows estimates of flexion and asynclitism. Is the vertex well flexed (the posterior fontanel is the key), hyperextended (the anterior fontanel is palpated more easily), or in midposition (neither fontanel predominates; both must be reached for)? A poorly flexed vertex infers that larger diameters of the vertex are presenting. It will take more labor time and work to complete the process.

Sutures of the vertex, coordinated with the fontanels, supplement the estimate of flexion of the vertex and the identification of the fontanels. The sagittal suture also adds information as to lateral flexion or asynclitism. For example, in a vertex with occiput transverse, a posterior or U position of the sagittal suture suggests to the examiner that the anterior parietal bone is presenting.

Molding and caput of the presenting part are also important clinical indicators of what is expected in the labor. At times caput may be present early in labor through a partially dilated cervix, particularly when membranes are ruptured. Molding connotes that the diameters of the vertex are changing in the fetal attempt to traverse the pelvis. Molding may take place above the ischial spines at higher pelvic stations in longer labors, or below the ischial spines after engagement occurs and during vaginal dilatation, or when descent of the vertex has been more rapid or has occurred earlier in labor. In general, in long labors molding takes place at higher stations, and in short labors time may be needed for the vertex to mold in order to traverse the vagina. Molding and caput, when felt during a difficult active or second stage of labor, suggests that the vertex is higher in the pelvis than it feels by palpation. In a protracted active-phase or a slow vertex descent during the second stage, the vertex feels lower than it actually is. Do not focus on the increasing caput and molding of the fetal vertex with progress in descent.

EXAMPLE OF CONFUSION IN ESTIMATING PELVIC STATION

A primigravid patient was experiencing a delay in descent during the second stage of labor. After 3 hours of full dilatation, the vertex, which had been at S+1 at 5 pm was felt to be at S+2 (based on five positive stations in the pelvis below the spines) at 8 pm, with an OP presentation.

Comment

Despite the station change, progress may still be arrested. The palpated descent may be increased molding and caput. The vertex is longer but the widest diameters are not lower. In an emergency or with the need to deliver this fetus rapidly, be concerned that this delivery may be more difficult than the position of the vertex suggests. The vertex may truly be comparable with a station 0 or even unengaged. Clinical events and judgment as to birth route dictate your next acts, but cesarean rather than midforceps or vacuum extraction should be carefully considered.

Stations of the Pelvis

Generally it is accepted that five stations should be used to define the depth of the pelvis. The midplane of the pelvis, as defined by the ischial spines and the theoretical bispinous plane, is called 0 station. The pelvic inlet is therefore estimated to be 5 cm above this line, and the reference is in minus (–) terms. The outlet is estimated to be 5 cm below this line and the reference is in positive (+) terms. Therefore, it is usual to estimate engagement at station 0 to +1 with crowning at station +5. Some clinicians use three stations instead of five, but this is discouraged. The five stations are estimated as a measurement in centimeters. These estimates become important in considering the application of forceps. This will be discussed in the chapter on forceps. As noted earlier, some clinicians use fundal pressure to determine whether the presenting part dips into the pelvis or between the ischial spines, and to predict adequate pelvic capacity. Although this is certainly a good omen, it is not always correct. Descent often takes place before labor for the primipara, and even more commonly takes place late in the active or second stage for the multipara.

High stations of the presenting part in early labor foreshadow longer labors but do not usually predict pelvic capacity. In latent labor findings, a station of S-4 rarely foreshadows "dystocia." Cesareans performed in latent-phase labor for dystocia result from inaccurate estimates of pelvic capacity by the physician. The cervix needs to dilate; then descent tests the pelvis.

Because estimates of pelvic capacity are always speculative, and because labor is not harmful, time to observe dilation and descent should be used before the labor is ended. In most instances, cervical dilatation will proceed whether or not descent take place. Referring back to the initial admission obstetrical examination, which should include the description of cervix and evaluation of the presenting part within the pelvis, as noted in Table 4.1, is the best way to measure progress.

Clinical Pelvimetry

Today few clinicians can describe the anatomy of the pelvis with its four bones, including the sacrum, the coccyx, and the two innominate bones (also known as the ilium, the ischium, and the pubis) and the pelvis lying above the iliopectineal line, with its muscular insertions (iliac muscles) running into the bony pelvis below it. For a more complete view of anatomy of the pelvis, refer to a standard anatomy text or a current volume of an obstetrical textbook.

Measuring Pelvic Capacity

In contrast to defining bones and muscle insertions, which are of interest but have little practical application, the length of the diagonal conjugate, the size of the sacrosciatic notch, the shape of the sacrum, the prominence of the ischial spines, and the splay of the pelvic side walls convey useful information and should be measured at the initial prenatal visit and again at the onset of labor if any abnormality is suspected. Relaxation of ligaments may result in greater measurements than those recorded early in pregnancy.

Estimating the diagonal conjugate is a very useful measurement. The term *estimate* is used with the understanding that the distance from the sacral promontory

Table 4.1   Obstetrical Examination

1. Dilatation of cervix (also its position: anterior, posterior, etc.)

2. Effacement of cervix (stated in percentage)

3. Presenting part (vertex, breech, other)

4. Position of fontanel (if both cannot be felt, think of the reason).
    When the head is not well flexed, a longer labor may be
    anticipated. Full flexion and extension must occur prior to most
    term births.

5. Station of presenting part in the pelvis (if the spines are
    prominent, note this)

to the underside of the symphysis pubis, as defined by the distance from your examining fingertip at the promontory, is stated to be about or greater than 11.5 cm. Usually, this measurement is adequate or longer than the examiner's finger may reach. If frequently performed on all patients, the repeated estimation of the diagonal conjugate allows the clinician to gain an experience estimating, not only possible inlet capacity, but also, as the finger traverses the hollow of the sacrum, the shape of the sacrum.

Can the head fit into the curve of the sacrum? This may be inferred if the sacrum is flat or knobby, thereby partially occluding the midplane and keeping the vertex high.

Are the spines so prominent that the vertex must rotate to an AP or oblique diameter before engagement can take place? Prominent spines suggest that a diameter other than the transverse diameter is necessary for engagement to occur.

Is the sacrosciatic notch wide? If so, expect more room in the posterior sagittal plane of the pelvis. The sacrosciatic notch is measured by moving the examining finger from the ischial spines, back along the sacrospinous ligament towards the sacrum. Once again, only after repeated attempts to make this estimate will the clinician gain sufficient experience to estimate size. In this case, the sacrosciatic notch is usually estimated to be between two and three finger-breadths (Fb) wide. A narrow ligament (<2 Fb) suggests a high arch with little space in the posterior aspect of the pelvis. A wide arch (>3 Fb) suggests a large posterior pelvis with more room for the vertex in this area of the pelvis.

It is difficult to estimate the pelvic sidewalls as the patient's muscle tension often confuses the measurement. It is more accurately measured during the patient's initial antepartum visit rather than during labor. In palpating the pelvic sidewalls, involuntary patient muscle contractions give the impression that the bony walls are convergent. In your mental picture of the pelvic capacity, attempt to separate the muscle tension from the true convergent pelvis, which is quite uncommon.

The final measurement is of the pelvic arch and the distance between the two ischial tuberosities. By placing two fingers under the pubic arch, the examiner can determine whether the shape of the outlet is narrow or wide. This is then confirmed by placing the fist between the two tuberosities. This examination, based on the distance across the fist, can confirm any narrowing of this outlet. A complete examination, including the above-mentioned measurements (diagonal conjugate, sacrosciatic notch, ischial spines, sacrum, and outlet), along with the clinical estimate of what may be expected for the labor, allows the clinician to estimate labor length and to identify potential problems. While these estimates may be inaccurate or change as labor progresses, they act as signposts along the way and encourage reevaluation and earlier intervention. For more detail, the reader may find that some of the older textbooks, such as that by Steer,[1] give excellent explanations of the pelvis and its clinical examination.

In a pregnancy following a cesarean for "dystocia," vaginally born siblings are often larger than their cesarean born predecessors. Therefore, it becomes apparent that despite the best clinical estimates, prediction for outcome will be only a first step towards a test of the pelvis, and only a trial of labor will determine the outcome.

X-ray Pelvimetry

Whether or not to order x-ray pelvimetry always arouses debate. It would appear that the fear of malpractice allegations may have reintroduced the dilemma. The dilemma is that in the absence of absolute pelvic contracture, the presenting part will flex, bend, mold, and work its way through this irregular passageway and delivery will take place. X-ray pelvimetry is not needed and adds little to patient management. The x-ray measurements are only estimates, and the numbers are far from exact. Because x-ray pelvimetry is infrequently used, both the persons taking the films and those reading the films confound the issues even further with their lack of knowledge. X-ray pelvimetry does not allow us to predict labor outcome. Obstetrical care has changed since the statement by Thoms,[2] in the preface to his text on pelvimetry, that during the previous 25 years all patients in labor in the clinical service at the Yale-New Haven Hospital had undergone an x-ray exam on admission.

It is therefore rare to perform x-ray pelvimetry for the vertex presentation. This examination may be performed for the breech presentation for two reasons. The first reason is to confirm vertex flexion and the absence of congenital anomalies, which can also be confirmed by ultrasonography or a flat x-ray film of the abdomen. The second reason is solely for protection so that after a difficult breech delivery, an x-ray pelvimetry examination can be shown as a part of the management decision should the result be less than anticipated.

Summary

1. The general history and physical examination, although shortened because of previous examinations, should be repeated at labor onset.

2. The obstetrical clinical evaluation consists of
   a. Observing the abdomen
   b. Palpating the abdomen
   c. Estimating cervical dilatation and vertex position
   d. Repeat clinical pelvimetry if necessary

3. Taken alone, each physical diagnostic task has limited value, but performed as a complete unit, adequate estimates of fetal size and pelvic capacity allow for more accurate predictions of labor length and labor outcome.

4. Clinical menstruation of the pelvis is best performed early in pregnancy and cannot be used as an absolute predictor of successful or unsuccessful vaginal birth.

5. X-ray pelvimetry adds little to labor management or estimates of pelvic capacity.

References

1. Steer CM. Moloys Evaluations of the Pelvis in Obstetrics, ed 2. Philadelphia, WB Saunders, 1959.
2. Thoms H. Pelvimetry. New York, Hoeber-Harper, 1956, p 9.

Chapter 5

The Latent Phase of Labor

Overview

In Chapters 5 through 8, the latent and active phases and the second stage of labor are reviewed. Dystocia is presented separately in Chapter 9. There is considerable overlap between phases and stages of labor, and in the therapeutic interventions use. Often, many of the same treatments are used in latent and active labor. In addition, it is sometimes difficult to distinguish the management of dystocia as a separate entity from the management of abnormal labor patterns. The reiterative process is used to provide simple, repeated guidance to the clinician, with the objective being to improve the understanding of the rationale for clinical care.

In the latent phase, cesarean delivery for such indications as failure to progress, cephalopelvic disproportion, or dystocia is most often inappropriate because the data for making those diagnoses are not available. Later, in active phase or the second stage of labor, when the duration of labor may be more accurately predicted, one is able to consider these diagnostic abnormalities in arriving at therapeutic decisions.

During the latent phase, decisions to terminate labor should, with few exceptions, be based on urgent maternal or fetal indications. In the presence of a nonreassuring fetal status, it may be prudent for the labor to be surgically terminated. Regardless of the stage of labor, in the presence of maternal hemorrhage, both maternal and fetal indications take precedence. Obviously, the degree of fetal or maternal compromise will influence these clinical decisions.

Objectives

At the conclusion of this chapter, the clinician should be able to

1. Define latent-phase labor
2. Diagnose the many factors affecting latent-phase labor

3. Describe management guidelines for latent-phase labor

4. Lower the incidence of cesareans in latent-phase labor

Latent Labor Defined

Contractions and Latent-Phase Onset

Latent labor onset is defined as the point at which the mother perceives regular contractions. To be certain that one is observing the latent phase, this must be followed by cervical dilatation as observed by the clinician.[1] An alternate approach defines labor onset only by observed cervical dilatation after the patient arrives at the hospital.[2] Neither of these definitions defines physiology or pathology, and it is arguable as to their validity. Either definition is acceptable as long as there is an understanding as to which system is being used. In this text, onset of the latent phase of labor is understood to begin with maternal perceptions of regular uterine contractions.

The clinical problem is to determine whether (or not) the patient who is experiencing contractions is really in labor. That question can only be answered by observation because it is cervical dilation, in the final analysis, that separates true labor from false labor.

In earlier studies at Cleveland Metropolitan General Hospital,[3,4] latent-phase labor lengths (in hours) were derived from time of onset of contractions, as noted by the patient, and were compared with the Friedman data, which accepts a similar definition. The results are remarkably similar.

In addition to the time of contraction onset, latent labor must be characterized by some observed cervical dilatation. No matter for how long contractions have been occurring, how frequently they may be felt or palpated by staff or visualized on a tocograph, and how distressing they may be for the patient, labor cannot be defined with certainty by uterine contractions alone. Dilatation must take place. An exception to that rule is the extremely uncommon condition of primary cervical dystocia, a condition in which the cervix is incapable of dilating because of previous cervical surgery and scarring.

EXAMPLE OF DIFFICULTY IN DETERMINING LABOR ONSET

On arrival at the hospital, a gravida I, para 0 was experiencing extremely painful contractions every 2 minutes. As noted on the tocograph, the contractions were bell shaped, with high peaks and poor return to the baseline. The vertex was floating; the cervix was 1 to 2 cm dilated in posterior position and 50% effaced. The fetal heart recording was normal. The diagnosis of possible placental abruption had been considered because of the severe maternal discomfort. The patient was observed for the next 2 hours with the obstetrician sitting at the bedside.

Comment

The diagnosis of possible abruption was later replaced by the diagnosis of false labor. With reassurance and maternal support (which was badly needed by the tense patient), the contractions changed in frequency and became more widely spaced, finally occurring about one each 10 to 15 minutes. The patient soon fell asleep. Five hours later, the patient had no contractions. In reviewing the previous events, it was felt that the patient was experiencing false labor.

No matter how impressive contractions may appear on the monitoring printout, contractions without dilatation cannot be interpreted as labor. In this typical example of false labor, the presence of the physician at the bedside helped to alleviate the patient's anxiety, with the subsequent disappearance of the uterine contractions. At first, all would have agreed the patient was in labor and fetal risk from a possible abruption was present.

Onset of Dilatation

Although regular contractions may signal the onset of the latent or active phases of labor, at the time contractions begin, neither patient nor physician can be certain that true labor is beginning. O'Driscoll and Meager[2] noted that in labor-room evaluations of mothers with cervices dilated less than 4 cm, 10% of the patients were eventually sent home because the diagnosis of active labor could not be confirmed.[4] One half of these patients soon returned in active labor and experienced early labor at home without harm to mother or fetus. For the remainder, the diagnosis of false labor was correct. O'Driscoll and Meager did not feel that taking more time to evaluate whether true labor had begun prior to initiating active labor management was a risk to either mother or fetus. Their study also demonstrated that even experienced physicians have difficulty making the diagnosis of true or active labor.

EXAMPLE OF INDUCTION DURING POSSIBLE LATENT PHASE LABOR (FIGURE 5.1)

A primigravida at 38 weeks of gestation appeared in the screening area for the third successive night. Because of her emotional distress, an induction of labor with oxytocin was attempted. On admission, the cervix was 1 to 2 cm dilated, 50% effaced, in midposition, with vertex at S-3. The fetus appeared normal in size. Eighteen hours after the oxytocin infusion was begun, the cervix was 3 cm dilated. For the first time, it was felt that the patient was in the latent phase of labor.

Comment

In this patient, labor was induced under unfavorable circumstances. As was predictable from the only partially effaced cervix, a long latent phase should have been anticipated. It

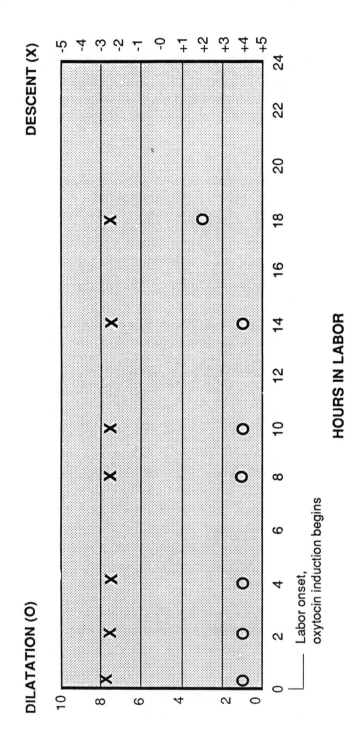

FIGURE 5.1

is this clinical situation that leads to patient and physician exhaustion, and what might have been avoidable cesarean deliveries. Eventually, if allowed to progress, this exhausted patient will not tolerate active and second-stage labor. Once again, interventions such as cesareans and forceps use will occur more frequently. As seen in Figure 5.1, this appears to be a problem labor, but it is only a long latent-phase induction.

An alternate management strategy could have been the use of adequate amounts of sedation and hydration, allowing the patient to sleep in the hospital overnight. Analgesics such as meperidine, rather than a barbiturate, are suggested since pain was part of the clinical picture.

As a general rule, the patient in the early latent phase of labor belongs at home. In the Cleveland study, less than 16.2% of patients who presented to the labor assessment area were admitted with evaluation exams of less than 3 cm cervical dilatation.[3] The key to the diagnosis of latent-phase labor is observed cervical dilatation. As Hendricks et al.[5] have stated, the cervix may dilate several weeks before labor begins. Thus, the antepartum nullipara or multipara with the cervix dilated at 1 to 2 cm is not uncommon, and 3 to 4 cm is not rare. In Table 5.1 note that at the time of admission for labor, the median dilation for nulliparous patients was 4 to 5 cm. If much of the latent phase of labor is spent at home, labor appears to be shorter to both the mother and obstetrician.

End of Latent Phase—Onset of Active Phase

The Friedman criteria for progress in the active phase of labor are widely accepted. In the nullipara, a cervical dilatation rate equal to or in excess of 1.2 cm/hr is considered active labor. In the multipara, the criterion for active labor is a cervical dilatation rate equal to or in excess of 1.5 cm/hr. This rate of cervical dilatation does not start at a specific dilatation. In an analysis of latent labor, 29% of patients reach 5 cm of dilatation before their dilatation rates conform to the Friedman dilatation rate of active labor. Conversely, other patients dilated more rapidly and had active labor-phase cervical dilatation rates beginning with as early as 3 cm of cervical dilatation.

If at term, with uterine contractions resembling a laborlike pattern in the presence of cervical dilatation, all patients should demonstrate an active-phase rate of cervical dilatation by the time they are 5 cm dilated. In other words, all patients should be "in active labor" by the time they reach 5 cm dilatation. If active-phase cervical dilatation rates are not present by the time the patient is 5 cm dilated, the obstetrician must begin to consider the initiation of treatment. The questions that should be asked include: Why hasn't an appropriate rate of dilatation yet occurred; What obstetrical interventions should be used to improve progress in labor?

Rather than set an arbitrary length to the latent phase of labor, Table 5.2 may be used to document mean latent-labor duration percentage of patients at dilations of 0 to 5 cm[3]. These average durations of the latent phase may guide the clinician to

Table 5.1 Dilatation of Patients on Admission[a]

Dilatation (cm)	% of patients
1	0
2	3.4
3	12.8
4	22.7
5	22.7
6	13.6
7	9.7
8	5.4
9	4.0
10	1.4
Complete	4.3
	100

[a]Normal patients with normal labors
Modified from Peisner Rosen,[3] with permission.

intervene when these limits are exceeded. In Friedman's descriptions, a prolonged latent phase is greater than 20 hours for the nullipara and greater than 14 hours for the multipara.[6] Neither number predicts abnormality of the active phase nor increased fetal morbidity. These numbers simply indicate that 90% of all women will have entered active labor by the end of the mean time period relative to dilatation at admission. From the Cleveland Metropolitan General Hospital data,[3] the mean length of latent labor for all patients was 6 hours and 49 minutes. However, this was a low-risk, normal population with amniotic membranes intact at labor onset.

In summary, the latent phase of labor ends at 5 cm dilatation or earlier if the rate of dilatation equals or exceeds 1.2 cm/hr for the nullipara or 1.5 cm/hr for the multipara. Early latent phase is best treated at home. Patients and physicians appear to perform better if the early latent phase of labor is not spent in a hospital labor room. The onset of latent phase labor may only be judged in retrospect after cervical dilation has been observed.

Ruptured Membranes and Latent Phase Labor

In the presence of ruptured membranes, the patient is often admitted to the hospital. In patients with ruptured membranes, prolapse of the umbilical cord and consequent fetal death is infrequent, about 1 per 2000 live births in term infants during labor.[7] This figure was obtained prior to the era of monitoring and applies to *all* labor, not only the situation of membrane rupture prior to labor.

Treatment following rupture of membranes without labor onset remains variable. At term with a favorable cervix (or after the 34th week at the Sloane Hospi-

Table 5.2   Mean Latent Labor Duration

Admission dilation (cm)	Mean h, min
0–2	9 h, 27 min
2–3	7 h, 46 min
3–5	5 h, 22 min

From Peisner and Rosen,[3] with permission.

tal for Women of the Presbyterian Hospital in New York City) many clinicians induce labor. If the cervix is not easily inducible, almost any pattern of care has been recorded in the literature—from no induction to induction at varying time intervals. Data proving efficacy for one consistent mode of treatment are not available. Cord prolapse and infection are the major concerns.

Prior to 35 weeks of gestation varied modes of treatment have been proposed, with no single approach being uniformly accepted. In the low-birthweight fetus, more clinicians tend to await labor onset rather than induce with oxytocin. In this population, fetal infection is more morbid.

Factors Affecting the Length of the Latent Phase of Labor

Cervical Dilatation

The cervical dilatation at the time of admission is the most accurate predictor of the remaining length of labor.[3,4] On average, the latent phase of labor will be 9 hours, 27 minutes if first seen at less than 2 cm dilatation. Latent phase will last 7 hours, 46 minutes if the patient is admitted at 2 to 3 cm dilatation. Beyond 3 cm of cervical dilatation, the average length of latent phase will be 5 hours, 22 minutes (see Table 5.2).

In a multivariate analysis of the known factors associated with the prediction of labor length, cervical dilatation was the most important variable when compared with parity, station, and status of the membranes.[3]

Station of Vertex

Descent of the vertex often takes place late in the active phase and continues during the second stage of labor. Many multiparas will not display vertex descent until full cervical dilatation takes place. Although most clinicians anticipate a more rapid labor progression when a vertex is deep in the pelvis (station +2 to +3), statistically, at onset of labor, station shows little predictive effect on the length of the latent phase.

Parity

Parity has little observed effect on length of latent phase. It accounted for about 1% of the length of latent phase in a statistical study attempting to define the relative importance of parity, dilatation, and station on length of labor.[3] This is in contrast to the second stage of labor, in which parity has a more obvious effect.

Maternal Age

The latent phase of labor is not influenced by maternal age. During labor, in the absence of maternal or fetal pathology, labor management should not be altered because of a maternal age factor. Statements such as, "This is a very important baby" or "This is a premium baby because of a history of infertility" should not influence clinical labor decisions. There are little data to suggest that maternal age (without observed pathology such as hypertension) should increase fetal risk or auger a more difficult labor. Similarly, infertility, once overcome, is not a labor management problem.

Rupture of Membranes During Latent Phase

The Cleveland Metropolitan General Hospital review of spontaneous and artificial rupture of membranes confirmed Friedman's earlier studies.[6,8] There was little effect of membrane rupture on labor length. The point to be made is that if it takes sophisticated statistical manipulations on large populations to show small effects, this information, although statistically correct, will not help the clinician's management choices in any individual case.

Guidelines for Artificial Rupture of the Membranes

If it is accepted that in the average patient membrane rupture does not contribute to the length of labor, when should membranes be ruptured?

1. Routine rupture of membranes is not indicated when labor is progressing satisfactorily. It adds little to the rapidity of cervical dilatation.

2. Artificial rupture of membranes (AROM) should be considered if labor is not progressing satisfactorily. Perhaps this will change the course of labor. This is not in conflict with the previous statement. In normal labors, AROM makes little contribution to the rate of cervical change. In slow or prolonged labor, the data have not been obtained that a helpful effect is possible, but clinical experience suggests it may be helpful.

   Note that the dilatation effect after membrane rupture is not immediate and may take time. Often, immediately following AROM, a small regression in cervical dilatation may take place before the vertex becomes well applied to the cervix.

3. Rupture of membranes may be performed in some instances of uncertain fetal status. It may be clinically helpful to know if meconium is present.

4. Rupture of membranes should be performed if internal fetal monitoring is needed and adequate monitoring information cannot be obtained from an external recording.

5. Rupture of membranes should be considered if uterine size is excessive. Note that too rapid contraction of the uterus after volume release may be associated with placental separation.

CASE EXAMPLE IN NULLIPARA WITH FAVORABLE CERVIX

A nulliparous patient at term is experiencing mild contractions every 7 minutes. The cervix is 3 cm dilated, 75% effaced, and the vertex is at S-1. The patient has a normal antenatal history, and external heart rate monitoring is unremarkable. It is the admitting physician's opinion that the patient is probably in early latent-phase labor. Since this is the first patient contact, progress in cervical dilatation has not yet been observed.

Option 1

Send patient home.
Her labor will have progressed further when she returns.

Option 2

Admit patient and observe.
This decision may be influenced by such factors as the level of the patient's apprehension and the geographic distance between her home and the hospital.

Option 3

Admit patient and induce or augment labor with oxytocin.
This decision is motivated by a clinical judgment that the patient's cervix is favorable for induction. Many clinicians would choose this option because at 3 cm and 75% effacement good progress might be anticipated.

Option 4

Rupture membranes and await dilatation or use oxytocin.
This decision is sometimes acceptable; however, once membranes are rupture, there is a commitment to maintaining monitoring, and completing labor. If the rupture of membranes has, at best, a small effect on labor length, why rupture the membranes to augment labor? If oxytocin is used, routine membrane rupture is not mandatory. It is always possible to discontinue the oxytocin if, despite the observed initial cervical dilatation, no progress occurs.

CASE EXAMPLE IN MULTIPARA WITH UNFAVORABLE CERVIX

A multipara at term with the vertex at S-3, cervix long posterior, and one fingertip dilated stated she had been experiencing contractions every 7 minutes for 24 hours. The fetal heart tracing over a 30-minute period was unremarkable. Occasional contractions were observed every 7 to 10 minutes.

Option 1

Send patient home.

This option is acceptable. If she and her spouse have not slept for the past 24 hours, perhaps more support may be offered.

Option 2

Admit patient and use sedation.

This is an acceptable option, and analgesia for pain may be provided. In the low-birthweight fetus, minimal medication is probably best.

Option 3

Induction or augmention with oxytocin.

In this case, it would be best to avoid this option. The unripe cervix augers a long latent-phase labor. At the extreme, it may take another 24 hours to reach active-phase labor. In this group of patients, cesarean deliveries are occasionally done because of the prolonged length of the latent phase. These patients represent difficult management problems.

Option 4

Rupture membranes and use oxytocin.

This plan is unacceptable for the same reasons noted in Option 3. Why look for trouble? At a later time it may be found that no cervical dilation has occurred or dilatation has not occurred at an acceptable rate. Eight or 10 hours will have passed, and the pressure to terminate labor by cesarean, often unnecessarily, will be present.

Although patients at term will frequently respond to oxytocin or to membrane rupture when the cervix does not feel inducible, the process is often lengthy and unpredictable. If there are medical indications to intervene aggressively, such as post-datism or toxemia, it no longer represents an elective situation. In most patients, there is no urgency to intervene during the latent phase of labor.

Six Management Strategies for Patients in the Latent Phase

There are six choices for patient care in latent-phase labor, and all six should be considered before a single approach is used.

Patience

If the average length of the latent phase is understood along with the knowledge that a 20-hour latent-phase labor is not rare, patience is a most important management tool. It had long been believed that a long latent phase does not predict dystocia, fetal compromise, or infant morbidity. However, in one recent study using multivariate linear logistic regression models,[9] a prolonged latent phase was independently associated with an increased incidence of subsequent labor abnormalities, need for cesarean delivery, depressed APGAR scores, and need for newborn resuscitation. However, despite this information, patience remains a useful conservative strategy.

Sedation and Analgesia

Meperidine or other narcotics are appropriate analgesics, particularly when pain is present and rest is needed. Rarely use barbiturates for these patients. Following narcotic analgesia, a 3- to 4-hour delay in cervical dilatation is not unusual. In the latent phase, the normally slow cervical dilatation may be prolonged further by medications. Avoid routine medication use in latent labor.

Regional Anesthesia (Epidural Anesthesia)

Regional anesthesia is frequently used in active labor. However, in latent-phase labor an epidural block should be limited to the unusually fearful patient or to the unusually painful labor. It is not unusual that following the initiation of an epidural block in the latent phase, labor will not progress until the anesthetic wears off unless oxytocin is instituted.

Oxytocin Use

Oxytocin is a common intervention in a prolonged latent-phase labor to shorten labor. If the latent phase is proceeding slowly (e.g., less than 1 to 2 cm dilatation has occurred following several hours of observation), an oxytocin infusion may be initiated. In an individual case, if this is an appropriate strategy, the response to oxytocin should be noted fairly rapidly. It should be noted, however, that studies from the Birmingham Maternity Hospital[10] suggest that it is possible for the cervix to contract in early labor. They suggest that this response may be the result of incomplete preparation of the cervix for the process of dilatation and that it is seen during what is recognized as the latent phase in those women in whom the cervix is uneffaced and undilated. The authors further suggest that it is this property of the cervix that may explain the relatively poor results obtained with the use of oxytocin in the latent phase of labor.

Artificial Rupture of Membrane (ARM)

Despite the fact that statistical analysis has revealed that ARM contributes little to progress in cervical dilation, it is a treatment option. Although engagement of the vertex may not be present, the head should be within the pelvis. Before rupturing the membranes, one should attempt to determine whether the presenting part will descend and be firmly applied to the cervix. At times, with a high vertex or a large vertex one can anticipate a slow descent. Pressure on the fundus during a vaginal examination may indicate the extent to which the vertex may descend. If the membranes are ruptured and the vertex does not become well applied to the cervix, the absence of a dilating wedge may impede cervical dilatation. This is another reason for a latent-phase cesarean, which might have been avoided if membranes had not been artificially ruptured. Shortly after membrane rupture, there may be actual regression in cervical dilatation.

It is not clear why in some cases following ARM dilatation is rapid and in other cases no effect is seen. If the dilating membrane wedge is removed and the vertex does not easily move against the cervix, it may necessary to wait until molding, flexion, and descent occur before further dilatation takes place.

Patient Position

Another treatment option is to change patient position. Allow patients to sit or lie in more comfortable positions. Ambulate the patient when possible. In the presence of an unremarkable fetal heart, and even in the presence of ruptured membranes (with the head well fit into the pelvis), try to increase patient comfort and do not limit activity. It is not easy for a patient to lay flat on her back (or side) for hours, awaiting progress in labor. A lounge area properly monitored by the obstetrical staff is appropriate for many patients.

If membranes are ruptured and the patient leaves the bed, intermittent monitoring by auscultation or doptone should continue. Although guidelines for auscultation during latent phase suggest monitoring every 30 minutes is acceptable, the choice may be to monitor more frequently during ambulation.

The etiologies for a prolonged latent phase are not known. The latent-phase labor treatments are derived from clinical experience. Many physicians agree that latent-phase labor sedation is overused, but at times sedation may be useful during labor.

Use of conduction anesthesia in latent-phase labor is controversial. The literature varies in describing outcomes. There may be a place for conduction anesthesia during the latent phase; however, the preference is to use oxytocin and to avoid epidural analgesia.

False labor is a difficult management problem. It is wise to keep the early laboring patient out of the hospital labor room when possible. Appropriate clinical judgment that assesses all the available strategies is recommended.

Cesareans and the Latent Phase of Labor

In a study of 2845 uncomplicated labors (i.e., no maternal or fetal emergencies)[3,4] at Cleveland Metropolitan General Hospital, 18 labors (.006%) ended in cesareans before the end of the latent phase of labor. It was clinical belief that no clinician, regardless of experience, was able to predict "dystocia" or "relative CPD" without a trial of labor. The only exception to this tenet was the rare instance of absolute cephalo-pelvic disproportion in the severely contracted pelvis. The need for an adequate trial of labor is a principle often restated in this text. There are no data to suggest that a trial of labor in the vertex presentation is harmful to the fetus, or conversely, that the fetus is healthier if born without labor.

The Need for Departmental Policy

Departmental policy should promote the following general statements:

1. Cesarean deliveries should rarely be performed during the latent phase of labor because of a diagnosis of dystocia.
2. Cesarean delivery in the absence of labor should rarely, if ever, occur because the obstetrician has made the clinical diagnosis that the fetus will not fit through the pelvis.
3. Cesarean deliveries should rarely be done without a trial of induction.
4. Cesarean deliveries should rarely be done in trial inductions before observed dilatation of the cervix.

The key word in statements 1 through 4 is *rarely*. There may be individual variations based on the fetal or maternal status.

Summary

1. The latent phase of labor begins with the onset of uterine contractions, as described by the patient, with progression of cervical dilatation observed by the clinician.
2. The latent-phase labor ends and active-phase labor begins when cervical dilation rates are 1.2 cm/hr for the nullipara and 1.5 cm/hr for the multipara.
3. At 5 cm of cervical dilatation, no matter how slow the cervical dilatation rate is, the latent phase of labor has ended and the active phase has begun.
4. Cervical dilatation at the time of admission most accurately predicts the length of labor.
5. Artificial rupture of membranes contributes little to normal progress in labor and should not be used as a routine management plan. It should be reserved for labors in which problems in the fetus, or of progress, may be present.

6. Six acceptable management strategies for latent phase labor are
   a. Patience
   b. Sedation or analgesia
   c. Regional anesthesia
   d. Oxytocin use
   e. Artificial rupture of the membranes
   f. Ambulation and position changes
7. Cesareans performed in latent-phase labor should rarely relate to labor abnormalities and should only be performed for maternal or fetal indications.

References

1. Cohen W. Friedman E. Management of Labor, Vol 2. Baltimore, MD, University Park Press, 1983, p 12.

2. O'Driscoll K, Meager D. Management of Labor, Vol 5. London, WB Saunders, 1980, p 25.

3. Peisner D, Rosen MG. The latent phase of labor in normal patients: A reassessment. Obstet Gynecol 1985;66:644–648.

4. Peisner D, Rosen MG. Transition from latent to active labor. Obstet Gynecol 1986;68:448–451.

5. Hendricks CH, Brenner WE, Draus G. Normal cervical dilatation pattern in late pregnancy and labor. Am J Obstet Gynecol 1970;106:1065–1082.

6. Friedman EA, Sachtleben MR. Amniotomy and the course of labor. Obstet Gynecol 1963;22:755–770.

7. Intrapartum fetal distress. In: Antenatal Diagnosis. Bethesda, MD, National Institutes of Child Health and Human Development, publication 79-1973, 1979, pp 67–68.

8. Rosen MG, Peisner DB. Effect of amniotic membrane rupture on length of labor. Obstet Gynecol 1987;70:604–605.

9. Chelmow D, Kilpatrick SJ, Laros RK. Maternal and neonatal outcomes after prolonged latent phase. Obstet Gynecol 1993;81:486–491.

10. Olah KS, Gee H, Brown JS. Cervical contractions: The response of the cervix to oxytocic stimulation in the latent phase of labour. Br J Obstet Gynaecol 1993;100: 635–640.

Chapter 6

Treatment of Latent-Phase Labor Abnormalities

Overview

Although all labor pattern problems encountered by the clinician cannot be completely reproduced in the form of clinical examples in this textbook, diagnostic and management routines are presented in this chapter, along with examples of patient care patterns. A series of questions are posed that should generally be addressed in the written note in the patient's chart. By following this approach, a process will develop that allows for logical clinical judgment and improved patient care.

Objectives

At the conclusion of this chapter, the clinician should be able to

1. Recognize abnormalities in patients in the latent phase of labor
2. Describe therapeutic interventions during latent-phase labor
3. Understand the range of acceptable treatment options
4. Conduct an adequate trial of labor designed to avoid unnecessary termination of labor in the latent phase (in the absence of fetal or maternal risk)

Six Diagnostic Steps for the Evaluation of Latent-Phase Labor

1. Define the components of latent-phase labor:
   a. Onset
   b. Interval
   c. End
2. Describe the antenatal history of the patient.
3. Evaluate the pelvis (passage).
4. Evaluate the fetus (passenger).

5. Evaluate the contractions (power).
6. Evaluate the labor history.

Six Therapeutic Interventions for Latent-Phase Labor

1. Patience (time is a treatment)
2. Ambulation
3. Sedation or analgesia (nonregional)
4. Epidural block
5. Use of oxytocin
6. Artificial rupture of membranes

The Six Diagnostic Routines with Examples

1. Define the Components of Latent-Phase Labor

Latent phase labor begins with the onset of maternal contractions until observed cervical dilation takes place, at a rate of 1.2 cm/hr in the nullipara and 1.5 cm/hr in the multipara. As noted in Chapter 3, if there is any doubt about the rate of cervical dilatation, at 5 cm the patient is in the active phase of labor. The normal duration of latent labor may be 20 hours in the nullipara and 12 hours in the multipara. For descriptive purposes, latent phase is divided into three parts: onset, interval, and end of latent phase.

Onset Component of Latent Phase

This diagnosis is often difficult to make. The best approach is to extrapolate back to contraction onset in order to identify labor onset. Without observed dilation, it cannot be stated with certainty that the patient is in the latent phase of labor. In the chart note, after your initial examination indicate that the patient *may be* at the beginning of latent-phase labor.

Interval Component of Latent Phase

You have *observed* that dilatation has taken place. However, the rate of dilatation has not exceeded 1.2 cm/hr (nullipara) or 1.5 cm/hr (multipara). If 5 cm of cervical dilatation has been reached, no matter how long the latent has been present, the patient should be treated as if she is in active-phase labor. On the other hand, if the rate of dilatation is consistent with active-phase labor, even if the cervix is only 3 or 4 cm dilated, the patient is considered to be in active labor. If progress during the interval phase is slow, interventions may be appropriate. The longer the interval portion of the latent phase, the more likely there will be a tired patient when active-phase labor begins.

End Component of Latent Phase

At least two vaginal examinations need to be performed confirming that the active-phase dilatation rate is not present or 5 cm dilation has not been reached. The reason for including "end" as a segment of latent phase is that if there is uncertainty, the patient should be treated as if in the active phase and intervention should be used if progress is prolonged.

EXAMPLE OF PRELABOR CERVICAL DILATATION

In an office examination, a nulliparous patient at 41 weeks of gestation was found to be 2 to 3 cm dilated and 80% effaced.

Comment

This cervical dilatation may have been present for a number of days to weeks. The key words are *observed active dilatation,* and this has not yet been confirmed. In this example, select a patient management approach based not on the belief that the patient is in labor, but rather on the basis of the gestational length of 41 weeks. A patient at 41 weeks of gestation with a favorable cervix may be considered an appropriate candidate for induction. In contrast, with the same findings at 34 weeks of gestation, the patient probably would have been sent home and encouraged to avoid activity for the next several weeks.

---

2. Describe the Antenatal History of the Patient

In the chart note, describe preexisting risks that may modify clinical judgment for the carrier, the passenger, and the passageway or birth canal.

3. Evaluate the Carrier

Review any maternal risks based on the mother's physical size, clinical pelvimetry, and social problems. Record important risks in the chart note.

EXAMPLE OF A CARRIER RISK

A 250 lb, 5-foot tall primigravida is evaluated in the admitting area. The cervix is 3 cm dilated and 60% effaced, and the vertex is floating above the pelvic brim. Fetal size by clinical estimate is judged to be above 8 lb.

Comment

This clinical picture should suggest the possibility of a problem in pelvic capacity. Labor should be allowed to progress in order test the pelvis. In most cases, these patients, although at risk for cephalo-pelvic disproportion, deliver vaginally. The outcome of this individual labor cannot be predicted with certainty. The chart note should describe maternal size as well as the fetal position and size. Ultrasonographic techniques may assist in predicting fetal weight more accurately.

4. Evaluate the Passenger

Review the evidence for fetal position and size. Assess the maternal abdomen first by palpation. Use Leopold's maneuvers, even when using the ultrasound machine.

EXAMPLE OF A PASSENGER PROBLEM

In a multipara with a family history of diabetes and a history of previous vaginal births of 8- and 9-lb neonates, the fetal size on examination is felt to be over 8 lb. The fetal vertex overlies the pubic symphysis. The cervix is 2 cm dilated and maternal diabetes is in good control.

Comment

The fetal size should, if possible, be additionally assessed by sonography to rule out macrosomia before considering active intervention. Some clinicians suggest that a 4500-g fetal size estimate warrants an automatic cesarean. This arbitrary definition is only an opinion and not universally accepted. Assessment of the entire clinical picture, including the carrier, the passageway, and the labor is required.

The patient's treatment should be individualized. Aggressive interventions, such as oxytocin use, are discouraged in these situations. In contrast, in the presence of good progress, such as seen with the vertex descending into pelvis, a labor trial should most often be allowed.

Ultrasound estimates of fetal size in the very low and very high birthweight ranges have the greatest margins of error. As noted, if labor proceeds spontaneously and the vertex descends in a normal manner, vaginal birth is very likely. In circumstances in which a very large baby is anticipated, many clinicians would not use oxytocin nor midforceps at a later time. If vaginal birth is to occur, it will most often occur spontaneously. Shoulder dystocia is increased in the greater than 4500-g fetus group. However, there is a need for the physician to exercise clinical judgment in the presence of a large fetus.

5. Evaluate the Forces of Labor

Describe the contraction pattern along with the observed cervical dilatation. Is this effective?

EXAMPLE OF A POSSIBLE CONTRACTION PROBLEM

In an otherwise normal term multipara, painful contractions every 4 minutes were observed for 3 hours without any change in cervical dilation. The cervix remained 2 cm dilated and 70% effaced. The vertex was floating and the fetal weight was estimated to be about 7 lb.

Comment

Latent-phase labor onset has not been confirmed despite the presence of contractions. Intervention might be considered.

Treatment with oxytocin is suggested in this example. A second acceptable choice would be to allow the patient to rest with the aid of analgesics. Rupturing the membranes at this time would commit the clinician to delivery, and it is not certain that the patient is in labor. The uterine contractions, although painful, appear not to have not been effective.

---

6. Evaluate the Labor History.

Is the patient in labor? Is progress defined? A major challenge in latent labor management is ruling out false labor. Once false labor is ruled out, the options include inducing a patient who is not in labor (depending upon the physical examination findings), augmenting poor progress in the interval portion of latent phase, or doing nothing and allowing the patient to go home.

EXAMPLE OF EARLY INTERVENTION IN LATENT-PHASE LABOR

A multiparous patient was observed to dilate from 1 to 3 cm during the first 3 hours in the labor room. For the next 3 hours there was no progress in cervical dilatation.

Comment

Because dilatation of the cervix had been observed, this patient is in the *interval* portion of latent labor. This latent-phase labor is progressing slowly. Therapeutic intervention should be considered. Several acceptable treatment choices include: oxytocin, medication, rupture of membranes, or patience.

EXAMPLE OF DIFFICULTY IN DIAGNOSING ONSET OF LATENT-PHASE LABOR

A normal multiparous patient at term, whose cervix is 60% effaced and closed, was observed for 3 hours without cervical dilatation. Contractions were moderate in strength, occurring every 5 to 7 minutes. There were no perceived maternal or fetal risks.

Comment

Doubt exists as to whether this labor has begun. Should this patient be induced? There is no medical indication for aggressive management. Therefore, treatment is based on clinical patient evaluation. In this clinical situation, judgment between clinicians may differ. This patient may be better served by returning home since it is often better to spend most of latent-phase labor at home.

The Six Therapeutic Interventions for Latent-Phase Labor

Treatment is usually based on previous evaluations. In order to do this, there should be an attempt to define the latent-phase labor, to evaluate the maternal and fetal backgrounds, and to evaluate the labor history. This leads to therapeutic choices, which include the following:

1. Patience
2. Ambulation
3. Sedation or analgesia (nonregional)
4. Epidural block
5. Stimulation with oxytocin
6. Rupture of membranes

Patience

Taking more time is an acceptable treatment for a nonprogressing latent phase labor patient. It is the physician's judgment as to whether patience or a more active form of intervention is needed.

EXAMPLE OF SEVERAL CORRECT THERAPEUTIC CHOICES DURING LATENT PHASE LABOR

A normal nulliparous term patient was seen in the labor screening room with the cervix 1 to 2 cm dilated, 60% effaced, and the vertex at S-3. Irregular but painful contractions every 7 minutes persisted.

Comment

Several choices for treatment in this patient are present. Individualize treatment choices in each situation. If the labor and delivery room is extremely busy at the time of evaluation, this may influence your choice. If the patient has been calling you repeatedly about contractions and false labor, this too will influence the choice.

1. Send the Patient Home

This choice would be acceptable. However, with painful contractions this may not be possible. Without pain, the low-risk patient belongs at home this early in the latent phase. In this case, in the presence of support persons, waiting in the hospital is acceptable. Remember, this is not the only choice, but it may meet with this patient's needs.

2. Ambulation

This treatment speaks for itself. It may be useful in any phase of labor but is used most frequently at latent-phase labor onset when there is uncertainty that latent labor is present.

3. Medication

Using medication in latent phase has been both damned and praised. When it is used, the clinician cannot predict what effect it may have on later progress. The clinician should anticipate a 2- to 4-hour interval of little or no progress. The choice between whether to stimulate with oxytocin or to be passive (ambulation, patience, medication) must be based on the clinician's judgment of the individual patient.

4. Use of Oxytocin

Oxytocin may give a relatively prompt response, documented by progressive cervical effacement and dilatation during the first several hours. If the cervix is poorly effaced, one should expect some delay before dilatation takes place. Cervical dilatation in the latent phase in the presence of oxytocin may not be evident for several hours, in contrast to active-phase oxytocin use, in which the response should usually be noted within the hour.

In general, the use of oxytocin is an excellent method to shorten the latent phase and to save the patients' energies for later labor, when strength will be important. A prolonged latent phase may lead to a tired patient during the active phase. To avoid this, one should often intervene earlier in the latent phase by using oxytocin. Electronically monitoring the frequency of uterine contractions and the fetal heart should be performed whenever oxytocin is used. If the contraction pattern and the fetal heart are within normal parameters, membrane rupture is not necessary when using oxytocin. Failure to make progress in the latent phase of labor, in the presence of intact membranes, allows the clinician to turn off the oxytocin and delay intervention.

EXAMPLE OF FAILURE TO MAKE PROGRESS FOLLOWING OXYTOCIN USE DURING LATENT PHASE

A normal primigravida at 39 weeks of gestation was seen in the screening area with a vertex presentation, cervix 2 cm dilated and 40% effaced. A decision was made to use oxytocin, but the clinician could not be certain that the patient was in latent-phase labor. After 4 hours of oxytocin, despite regular uterine contractions every 3 minutes, no progress, as defined by cervical dilation, was noted.

Comment

Since the amniotic membranes were not ruptured, there is more flexibility in the next choices. If the fetal monitoring records are normal, the oxytocin may be stopped and the patient either sedated or sent home when contractions cease. As an alternate treatment, the membranes may be ruptured. A long latent-phase labor may be anticipated.

Membrane Rupture

This is an active intervention at this time. In the absence of fetal indications, it is less acceptable. At 1 to 2 cm dilatation and a high vertex presenting, if membranes are ruptured, a long induction can be expected with no possible conservative discontinuation.

EXAMPLE OF LATENT-PHASE LABOR INTERVENTION FOR PATIENT NEED

A multiparous patient at term was seen in the screening room. Examination revealed the cervix to be 1 to 2 cm dilated, 60% effaced, vertex at station S-3, and with a normal fetal and maternal antenatal history. For the previous two nights, the patient had little sleep and was obviously exhausted.

Comment

This patient needs rest. Do not expect a short labor. If pain is the problem, medicate appropriately with a narcotic. If pain is not the major problem, perhaps a mild analgesic would be sufficient. The family should be encouraged to support this approach. The auditory portion of the fetal monitor should be turned down or, alternately, a low-risk patient such as this one, need not be monitored. Do not hesitate to remove the abdominal straps and monitoring devices to make the patient more comfortable.

As noted in Chapter 3, AROM is less routinely suggested for use in the management of labor. It does not add to rapid cervical dilatation. There is little evidence to warrant the routine use of this treatment. Use membrane rupture with caution and only perform ROM when committed to completing an already established labor. Most membranes rupture spontaneously in normal labor. The rate of cervical dilation is often more rapid following spontaneous rupture of membranes (SROM) rather than AROM.

EXAMPLE OF A MANAGEMENT PROBLEM FOLLOWING AROM DURING LATENT PHASE

A normal nullipara noted contractions every 5 minutes for a period of 2 hours. The vertex was at S-0 and the cervix was 2 to 3 cm dilated. The fetal weight was estimated to be average and the pelvis estimated to be adequate. Because she was at station 0, it was elected to rupture the membranes. Despite the favorable cervix, dilatation did not occur. The vertex was now poorly applied to a 2 to 3 cm floppy cervix, with no observed change during the next 4 hours.

Comment

Nothing but trouble was gained by the membrane rupture. Now the only acceptable choice left for the clinician is to use oxytocin. Eventually in this labor (if the latent phase lasts 12, 18, or 20 hours) there will be some concern about the length of time of the ROM, and concern about infection will be added to the management problems. When AROM works, it is great. When it does not, it is a serious problem. Since this is often unpredictable, avoid rupturing membranes early or unnecessarily. The later in labor AROM is performed, the fewer problems will be encountered.

Cesarean

As stated previously, the use of the abdominal birth route as a treatment choice in latent labor should be uncommon. In many instances the selection of this intervention may reflect failure to correctly recognize that latent labor (onset) was not present. Pelvic capacity is not adequately tested by terminating labor with a cesarean during latent phase. In subsequent pregnancies, when discussing the reasons for their cesareans, these patients may recount labors described as 1 or 2 days in length. Yet the clinician can not be sure they were in labor.

Cesareans are performed in latent-phase labor for maternal or fetal indications. These indications may include hemorrhage, infection, fetal distress, and unusual fetal size or presentation.

Reviewing the Format for Analyzing and Treating Latent-Phase Labor

Asking and answering the following questions will provide a general format for a diagnostic process.

Diagnostic Process

1. Is the patient in latent labor? Yes __ No __
2. What is the phase of latent labor? Onset __ Interval __ End __
3. Are there background factors or concerns for the carrier, the passenger, the forces? Yes __ No __
4. Describe the obstetrical findings including contractions, dilatation of the cervix, and station of vertex.
5. Summary statement. The therapeutic choices follow as an outcome of the diagnostic process.

Therapeutic Choices

In your chart notes document the intervention and the time it was instituted.

1. Patience
2. Ambulation
3. Sedation or analgesia
4. Epidural block
5. Use of oxytocin
6. Rupture of membranes (cesareans are rarely appropriate here).

Diagnostic steps 1 through 5 are often routine parts of patient notes. The therapeutic interventions may take place in varied sequences, depending on clinical progress. *Time* is used to describe the start and finish of an intervention. The program is easily correlated with the graphic labor curves. Either the effect is seen or the effect is not working. Time for effect of the intervention lets the clinician know when to move on. With medication one should provide more time before intervening again; the effects may take hours. If oxytocin is used, more rapid change may be anticipated, often within the hour.

EXAMPLE OF LATENT-PHASE DIAGNOSIS AND TREATMENT

History

On admission, a healthy 28-year-old G3 P2 at 41 weeks gestation stated that her contractions had begun 12 hours earlier. At the time of admission the contractions were felt to be every 5 to 7 minutes and moderately painful. The patient's membranes were intact. On abdominal examination, the fetus was average in size, with the back on the left and the vertex unengaged. On vaginal examination, the vertex was LOT, station –3, cervix 1 to 2 cm dilated, posterior, 60% effaced, and soft. The patient's antepartum course was unremarkable, and her clinical pelvimetry was adequate (Fig. 6.1).

Diagnostic Plan (Chart Note)

We are uncertain that the patient is at the onset of latent labor. Although contractions began 12 hours earlier, there is no labor diagnosis yet. The mother has had a unremarkable antepartum course with normal clinical pelvimetry; the fetus is of average size and without evident risk.

12 h of contractions pass

Uncertain labor diagnosis exists

Patient is admitted to the hospital

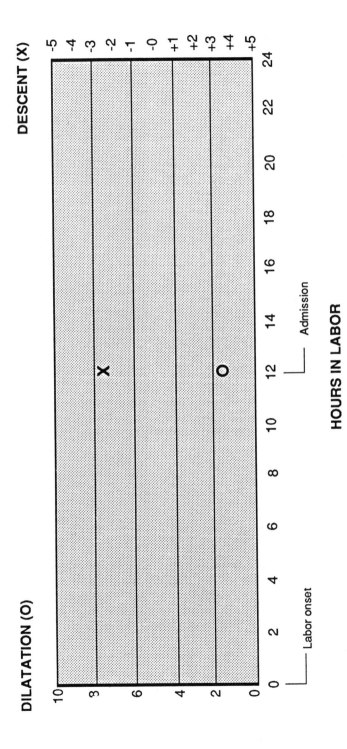

FIGURE 6.1

Write the Therapeutic Plan in the Chart

The choices include patience, ambulation, medication, epidural block, oxytocin, AROM, or cesarean.

Patience

This is the least aggressive mode of therapy. The patient has not been in hospital long enough to make a diagnosis. Many would choose to observe her progress for about 2 hours. Is it possible to send this patient home? Certainly, if this is acceptable to her.

Ambulation

At the end of a stated time period, if nothing changes while in the hospital, plan a new therapy. A time of 1 or 2 hours is more than sufficient for a patient to ambulate.

Medication

This is acceptable if pain is a major problem or if this patient is tired and needs rest. Even if in latent-phase labor, expect a delay of at least 2 to 4 hours in cervical response with dilatation. In this patient, pain does not appear to be a problem. The less medication used in latent-phase labor, the fewer confounding factors labor presents.

Epidural Block

This is unacceptable at this time. It is uncertain as to whether or not this patient is in labor. If used in the absence of observed cervical dilation, the need for oxytocin will soon follow. If used, it will need to be continued for many hours.

Oxytocin

This is less acceptable as a long labor is expected (cervix 60%). Why induce in the face of a long labor?

AROM

This is unacceptable at this time. There is no medical reason why this patient must deliver today. Once the membranes are ruptured there is a commitment. If delivery is the choice, the use of oxytocin is a more realistic option.

Cesarean

This is not an acceptable intervention. It is not known whether labor will fail (see Fig. 6.2).

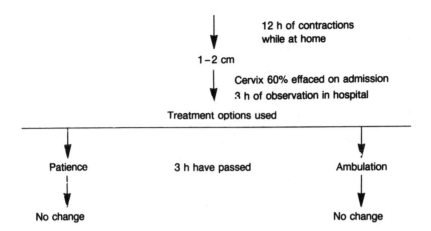

This patient may still be sent home or sedated and observed. If sent home, she may soon return in active labor. Nothing is lost. If sedated, she may wake up in active labor and nothing is lost. If no change occurs after sedation, this patient still may be sent home or labor stimulated with oxytocin. During the observation period, the patient should know her physician's opinion that she may not be in labor and that she may be sent home.

This patient was given 100 mg of meperidinedine intramuscularly for rest (see Fig. 6.3).

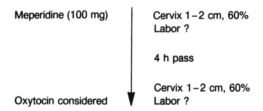

It is clear that this patient is not in labor. It must be understood that persisting means the patient is being induced. Labor is not being augmented since there is no labor. Dilatation has not occurred; therefore, the diagnosis of labor cannot be made. You may still stop this therapeutic trial after the use of oxytocin. It is a judgment that will vary among physicians.

This example illustrates the very common problem of uncertain labor onset. Treatment must be carefully evaluated in order to avoid creating new problems. At any point that intervention produces, cervical dilatation, therapeutic interventions

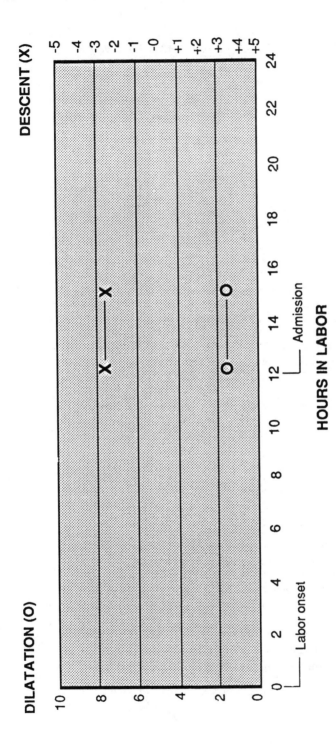

FIGURE 6.2

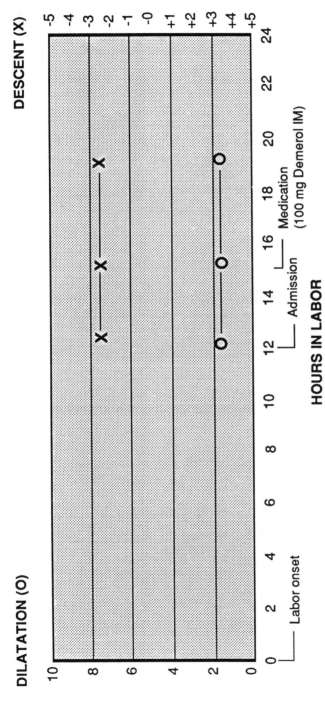

FIGURE 6.3

for management of latent-phase labor may be continued. When these patients are sent home, their management is simplified. In the hospital, patient care is more complicated because the clinician is more prone to "do something." However, generally, cervical change does occur. In the described patient, after 16 to 24 hours of living through the "possibility of labor," the physician's decision making often offers a commitment to persist to delivery. In cases such as this, the frequently occurring problem is false labor. It is important to rule out other confounding problems, such as genitourinary infections, placental abruption, gastrointestinal infections, and emotional distress. In the circumstances of a mother with fetal or maternal risks, the diagnosis would have altered the therapy and perhaps management would have become more aggressive (i.e., hospitalization, induction, or delivery would have been considered).

EXAMPLE OF LATENT-PHASE DIAGNOSIS AND TREATMENT

History

A 21-year-old multigravida at 39 weeks of gestation with a unremarkable antepartum history and inadequate clinical pelvimetry was admitted to the labor unit. She was found to be 3 cm dilated, 90% effaced, vertex at station −1 in the LOT position, with irregular uterine contractions that had begun 3 hours earlier. Her membranes were intact. The patient felt increasing pelvic pressure and back pain (Fig. 6.4).

Diagnostic Plan (Chart Note)

Latent labor onset or interval cannot be documented. Cervical dilatation is present but progress has not yet been observed. The mother and fetus appear unremarkable. Since the mother is at term with the cervix 3 cm dilated and 90% effaced, she could easily be induced. Her antepartum course was normal.

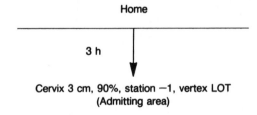

Home

3 h

Cervix 3 cm, 90%, station −1, vertex LOT
(Admitting area)

Therapeutic Plan

Patience

This is still possible, but other options may be more acceptable.

Ambulation

This, too, is still possible, but as in the patience option above, other options may be more acceptable.

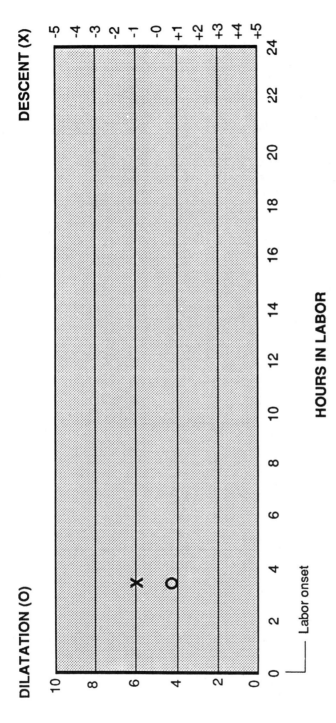

FIGURE 6.4

Medication

This therapy is not needed. Pain has not been a major symptom.

Epidural or Regional Block

This is not a usual therapeutic choice in the presence of an easily inducible cervix unless the patient is extremely tired.

Oxytocin

This is the procedure of choice. The oxytocin can be turned off in 4 to 6 hours if nothing happens. At times, even when it seems that the cervix will dilate, it may not. However, it is anticipated that dilatation will take place in this example.

AROM

This is not a preferred choice. Although AROM may be followed by contractions, the physician is committed to pursue the labor to delivery. In this case, there is no need to be committed to labor completion at this time.

Cesarean

This is not a choice at this stage (see Fig. 6.4).

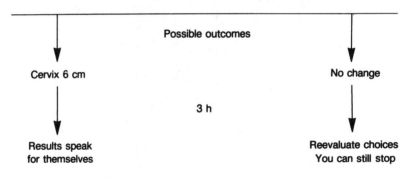

Course continues

(Cervix 3 cm, 90%, −1, OT)
Oxytocin was used for 3 h

Possible outcomes

Cervix 6 cm   No change

3 h

Results speak   Reevaluate choices
for themselves   You can still stop

Delivery will soon take place

Course

The patient rapidly dilated and entered the active phase of labor. If no change had occurred in 6 hours, the next choice might have been to medicate and rest the patient, then try again the next day, or await the onset of spontaneous labor. Membrane rupture commits to an inevitable course, and despite the favorable cervix and the fact that in cases such as this labor will generally follow AROM, it does not always happen. There appears to be an increase in the diagnosis of dystocia as an indication for cesareans. Some of this increase in the diagnosis may be due to unnecessary interventions in the term patient who is not in labor.

EXAMPLE OF ACTIVE INTERVENTION IN LATENT-PHASE LABOR

A 38-year-old multipara at 42 weeks gestation, with a normal antepartum course and adequate clinical pelvimetry, had a reactive nonstress test 48 hours earlier. She was first seen in the labor screening room with blood pressure 130/80, normal physical and laboratory findings, and a fetus of average estimated weight in a vertex presentation in the ROT position at S-3. The cervix was noted to be 2 cm dilated and 40% effaced. The amniotic membranes were intact and contractions had been present every 15 minutes for 2 hours.

Diagnostic Plan (Chart Note)

Although labor onset is still uncertain, there is increased risk because of a borderline elevated blood pressure and increased gestational length. Based on these clinical findings, a trial with oxytocin should be attempted. The chart note should describe the findings and the reasons for therapy.

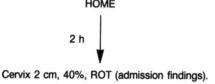

HOME

2 h

Cervix 2 cm, 40%, ROT (admission findings).

Therapeutic Plan (Chart Note)

Patience

This is probably an unlikely approach. A more aggressive approach at a reasonable hour, or with a rested patient, is indicated for mother and fetus.

Ambulation

This approach is not recommended. The clinical findings have increased the risk factors, and the fetus should be delivered as expeditiously as possible.

Medication

Pain or exhaustion is not the problem.

Regional Block

Similar to the medication option above, this is not indicated.

Oxytocin

This therapy is the intervention of choice. If progress occurs, delivery will take place before the risk factors have had an opportunity to become more severe. If progress does occur, and the fetus tolerates without evidence of distress what is in effect a prolonged contraction stress test, the new information will help in the management of the patient. In the presence of contractions, this would suggest that there is no deprivation of fetal oxygenation, which sometimes is a concern with post-term pregnancies, particularly with blood pressure elevation.

AROM

There would be no need to commit to an immediate delivery. It would be helpful to document the amount of amniotic fluid on ultrasound. A decreased amount of fluid might suggest the possibility of post-maturity syndrome. The presence of meconium along with the absence of amniotic fluid would probably prompt one to pursue delivery more aggressively and perhaps perform AROM.

Cesarean

This is not anticipated and would be a misuse of the information at this point in time. Even if the induction choice results in a long labor, there is no sign of fetal compromise (Fig. 6.5).

If, instead of response to oxytocin, no dilatation occurs, the physician has a more difficult therapeutic dilemma. Multiple options remain as long as the mother's clinical state does not deteriorate.

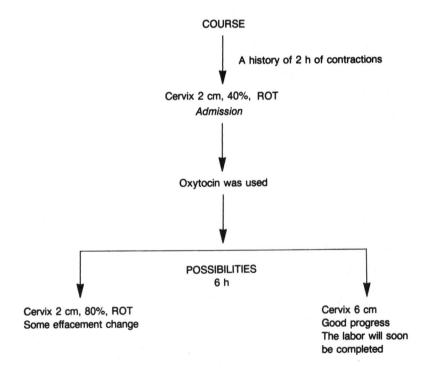

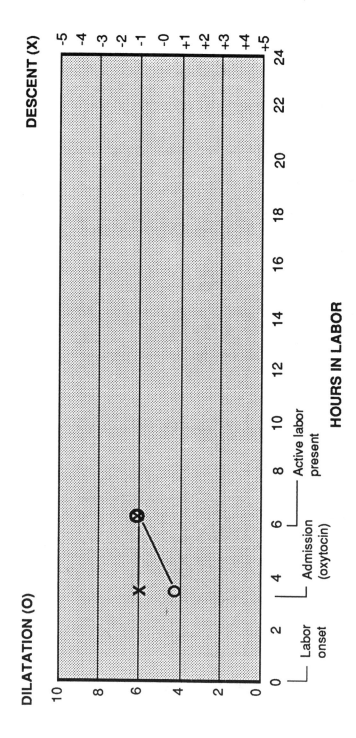

FIGURE 6.5

Therapeutic Choices if No Dilatation Has Occurred

Oxytocin

The clinician may continue as before. This labor may take 20 hours. Be prepared for a long labor, which is acceptable, in the absence of fetal distress.

Medication

No reason to use this yet. The patient has not expressed a need for pain relief.

Regional Block

If the patient needs a regional block due to pain, tension, or fatigue, then use it. In this case it is not an obvious need. This treatment can be used in association with oxytocin to make the patient more comfortable. However, it is more acceptable to use regional block after labor is well established.

AROM

AROM is a possible choice, but in view of the cervix, wait unless a change in fetal or maternal condition warrants a more aggressive approach. For example, if at any time monitoring information is technically poor or confusing with regard to fetal condition, an option may be to rupture the membranes. As noted previously, in the presence of good quality recordings, it is not necessary to rupture membranes in order to begin internal monitoring, even if oxytocin is being used.

Cesarean

This is acceptable in the presence of non-reassuring fetal heart rate recordings.

These examples of latent-phase labor abnormalities have been presented in terms of diagnostic evaluations and therapeutic plans. The key is a logical and organized assessment of the clinical situations. All available information should be used in the evaluation of the patient. All treatment programs should be considered. The interventions described encourage flexibility of choice and the use of patient care options, that do not necessarily compel completion of labor unless the decision becomes mandatory because of new patient risks.

Summary

1. When the patient is first seen on hospital admission, the chart note should

   a. Define the latent phase

   b. Describe the patient's early pregnancy history

   c. Evaluate the pelvis (passage)

    d. Evaluate the passenger (fetus)

    e. Evaluate the forces (power)

    f. Evaluate the labor history

2. The six clinical treatment choices available during latent phase include:

    a. Patience

    b. Ambulation

    c. Medication (sedation or analgesia)

    d. Epidural block

    e. Use of oxytocin

    f. Artificial rupture of membranes

3. Therapeutic options or combinations of therapeutic options may be used in a variety of sequences. If possible, avoid epidural block in early latent-phase labor.

4. Avoid interventions such as AROM in early latent-phase labor unless there are specific compelling reasons to do so.

5. Cesareans in latent-phase labor should only be performed for documented maternal or fetal risks.

6. Cesareans in latent-phase labor because of failure to progress should be very rare and may indicate the obstetrician's failure to adequately allow an appropriate trial of labor.

Chapter 7

Active Phase of Labor

Overview

If there is uncertainty as to when the latent phase has been completed and active labor has begun, confusion is added to the conduct of labor. The problem for the clinician is to understand when the active phase of labor has begun and the latent phase has ended. During active-phase labor more rapid interventions are required. Each change in a labor phase sets off a different series of clinical expectations. But even during active-phase labor, patience by the clinician to allow time for labor to progress is a primary treatment. In the absence of fetal risk or fetal distress, labor can often go "a little longer" before a decision to end it is reached. If about 28% of the cesarean birthrate is associated the diagnosis of "dystocia," then better understanding of active-phase labor management may lower the cesarean birthrate.[1]

Definitions for durations of latent phase, active phase, and second stage of labor are derived from averaging the lengths of labor of individual patients. It is harder to define the expectations of the birth process taking place during latent- and active-phase labor than during the second stage of labor. For example, in the labor of some patients vertex descent is already present early in labor. For most patients vertex descent is less common during the latent phase, more common during the active phase, and most common during the second stage of labor. Vertex descent and pelvic capacity are difficult to predict without an adequate trial of the active and second stages of labor.

Objectives

At the conclusion of this chapter, the clinician should be able to

1. Define the three parts of active-phase labor.
2. Complete chart notes to document the patient's course.

3. Use graphs for visual descriptions of active labor.
4. Understand the relationship of vertex descent to the active phase of labor and to the second stage of labor.
5. Understand all the therapeutic interventions for active-phase labor.
6. Understand the relationship between the end of active-phase labor and the onset of the second stage of labor.

Cervical Dilatation and Onset of the Active Phase

As noted in the previous chapter, about 50% of patients in labor are already dilating at rates greater than 1.2 or 1.5 cm/hr at 4 cm of cervical dilatation. Almost 90% of all patients have reached this rate of dilatation by 5 cm.[2] All patients should be considered to be in active-phase labor at 5 cm of cervical dilatation. The change in cervical dilatation rate from the slow latent phase to the rapid active phase is defined as the accelerative portion of active-phase labor. A slow accelerative phase may need an intervention such as augmentation.

EXAMPLE OF SLOW ACCELERATION DURING THE ACTIVE PHASE (Figure 7.1)

A primigravida, whose contractions began at 7 pm the previous evening, was 4 cm dilated at 7 am when first seen by the clinician. At 9 am the cervix was 4 to 5 cm dilated and in ROT position. At 11 am she was 5 cm dilated.

Comment

While this is not an arrest, the rate of dilatation is slow. Although the rate of dilatation suggests that this is still latent phase, according to the 5-cm rule the patient is in active labor and should be treated as if this is a protraction of the active phase. The slow dilatation of the cervix may need intervention. The chart note should describe whether there are any fetal problems in position, station, or size. Are contractions adequate? Is the mother exhausted or in a great deal of pain? The description in the patient's chart helps to formulate treatment. In order to avoid patient exhaustion, it is necessary to act early in treating this type of labor.

Charting Active-Phase Dilatations

As previously explained, the labor graphs used in this text are based on the Friedman curves.[3] A different charting method is a straight-line progression of labor rather than a curve with different slopes of cervical dilatation. The active management protocol of the National Maternity Center states that cervical dilatation

86

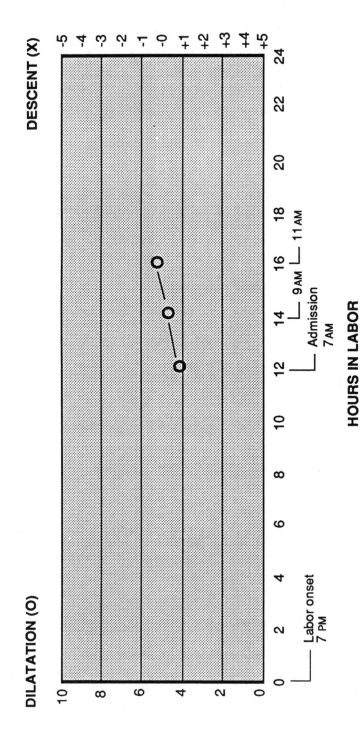

FIGURE 7.1

rates of 1 cm/hr should be expected. Oxytocin is used for primigravidas if this rate is not reached or maintained.[4] This graphic method is not derived from actual labor experience but is more easily understood.

In contrast, the Friedman graph uses rates of cervical dilatation and descent of the vertex derived from patient measurements, and the plotted curve has several slopes (Fig. 7.2).[3] In this text the model Friedman curves for cervical dilatation or vertex descent are not superimposed on the decision; however, too often deviation of a patient's cervical dilatation or descent rate from the classical labor pattern encourages the clinician to end labor. It is preferable to plot the patient's progress in labor and thus visualize whether progress is continuing. Intervention should occur only when progress is unacceptable. Deviation from an expected labor curve does not indicate an abnormality but represents a caution to the physician to reevaluate the patient. Too often the presence of a number is taken as an absolute. Each laboring patient is unique, and her labor must be assessed based on her situation and not because she fails to fit a predetermined average curve.

On the other hand, an elevated patient temperature warrants investigation, diagnosis, and treatment. Being aware of the event is important; flexibility of treatment is the art of obstetrics.

The Three Parts of Active Labor (Figure 7.2)

A–B Accelerative: A slow rate change or transition from latent to active

B–C Maximum slope dilation: A rapid rate change

C–D Decelerative: A slowing in active phase until molding, descent, or rotation takes place and second stage begins

Accelerative Phase

At the transition from latent- to active-phase labor, the cervical dilatation rate increases. This is seen in Figure 7.2 between points A and B. When there is movement from a slower to a more rapid rate of cervical dilation, the patient's labor chart reflects this with an abrupt upward change in the slope of the line. This portion of the graph describes the *accelerative phase* of active labor. There may be confusion as to when latent labor ends and active labor begin; that is why 5 cm is arbitrarily selected to define the transition.

Many patients are in the active phase of labor, as defined by their rate of cervical dilatation, before 4 cm dilatation is reached. These patients may dilate the cervix more rapidly and earlier, but they are rarely problem cases.[2]

Maximum Dilatation Phase

Cervical dilatation usually continues rapidly throughout most of the active phase. This is seen in Figure 7.2 between points B and C. The more vertical slope defines

88

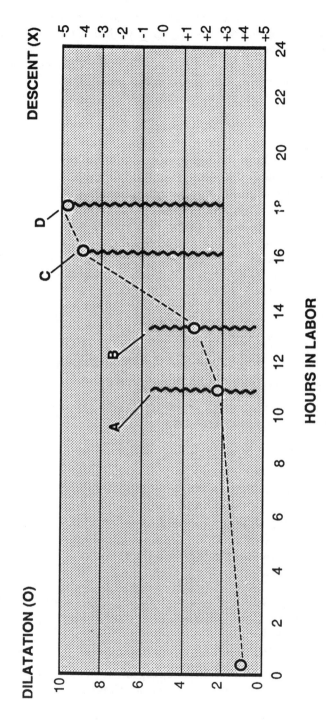

FIGURE 7.2

the *maximum dilatation phase*. The general rate of dilation of the cervix in active phase is 1.2 or 1.5 cm/hr, depending on parity (nullipara or multipara). It is important to plot the laboring patient's progress in the record. By plotting the progress, the clinician is made more aware of the actual pattern of progress than from relying on recall alone. However, the clinician's judgment should not be limited by reliance on the classic picture of the patient's progress. As noted earlier, 1 cm dilatation is an acceptable rate of change each hour. In this range, progress is continuous and there is little reason to intervene. The key word is *continuing* progress. If the patient is not continuing to progress, then a clinical diagnosis of a protraction or an arrest should be considered.

The diagnosis "Failure to Progress" has become very popular in this situation and is becoming a common pre-cesarean delivery diagnosis. Failure to continue progressing may be a precursor to cephalo-pelvic disproportion or other problems. However, it is a diagnosis of exclusion; thus, the clinician must evaluate all factors involved in labor and consider other treatments, which will be discussed in more detail later before moving to a cesarean delivery.

Decelerative Phase

The rate of cervical dilatation may slow as it approaches complete dilatation (see Fig. 7.2, between points C and D). The presence of a rim of cervix or a lip of cervix often persists longer than expected. Although the existence of the decelerative phase may not be seen in all patients, the decelerative phase may occur. It is more often seen in non–occiput-anterior vertex presentations. The occiput posterior or transverse vertex may not reach full dilatation until some descent and some rotation of the vertex occurs. In these positions the disappearance of the remaining cervix takes longer, and this time interval becomes the decelerative phase. In some patients it is expected that there may be a slowing of cervical dilatation as the vertex begins to descend, rotate, flex, and mold prior to the second stage of labor. This slowing is also normal.

Protractions and Arrests of Cervical Dilatation

Protractions and arrests in the active phase of labor have already been mentioned. Protractions and arrests have been defined by Cohen and Friedman[4] (Table 7.1), and the incidence of the problems has been described by Bottoms et al.[7] (Table 7.2) from the Cleveland data. This information is useful and helps to provide terms to describe the labor. It also provides guidelines for determining when labor deviates from the expected course and when interventions should be considered. The recognition of a protraction or an arrest is more easily diagnosed if the labor is graphed (Fig. 7.3).

A summary of labor abnormalities at Cleveland Metropolitan General Hospital

Table 7.1   Protractions and Arrests of Cervical Dilatation

	Nulliparas	Multipara (%)
Protracted active-phase dilatation	Maximum slope of dilatation of 1.2 cm/hr or less	Maximum slope of 1.5 cm/hr or less
Prolonged deceleration phase	Deceleration phase duration of 3 hr or more	Deceleration phase duration of 1 hr or more
Secondary arrest of dilatation	Cessation of active-phase progression for 2 hr or more	

After Cohen and Friedman,[4] with permission.

was derived from a data set of station and dilation recorded in the chart during labor. Table 7.2 reviews these data.

Assessment of Dilation in the Active Phase

Defining the three parts of active-phase labor will often be helpful in determining an individual patient's progress. During active-phase labor, a vaginal examination usually should be performed every 2 hours. If dilation is not increasing at about 1 cm/hr, reassess the clinical situation because progress of less than 1 cm/hr may not be satisfactory. The term *may* is used because it implies judgment for each individual patient. It is best not to set rigid limits for interventions.

When the cervical dilation rate falls to less that 1 cm/hr, the clinician needs to be aware of the rate in order to confirm a labor diagnosis. A judgment can then be made as to whether intervention is what a laboring patient needs. There may not be a need to intervene. In contrast, if three consecutive hourly examinations document an arrest of dilatation, it becomes necessary to consider several medical interventions.

EXAMPLE OF PROTRACTION IN THE ACTIVE PHASE (see Figure 7.3)

At term, in a normal pregnancy of a G3 P2 mother, the cervix was 7 cm dilated and the vertex was at station 0 in the ROA position at 9 am. At 10 am the cervix was 7 to 8 cm dilated and the vertex was still at station 0. At 11 am the cervix was 8 cm dilated with no change in station.

Comment

This is not a phase arrest. According to our expectations, the maximum slope of dilatation should have taken place, but it did not. This active phase of labor is protracted. It is time to

Table 7.2   Abnormal Labor Patterns[a]

Nullipara(%)		Multipara (%)
>21 hr (3.6%)	Prolonged latent phase	>14 hr (4.2%)
<1.2 cm/hr (25.6%)	Protracted active phase	Dilatation <1.5 cm/hr (16.2%)
No change for 2 hr (3.6%)	Secondary arrest dilatation	No change for 2 hr (6.8%)
Dilatation <1 cm/hr (10.4%)	Protracted descent	Dilatation <2 cm/hr (4.5%)
No change for 1 hr 5.8%	Arrest descent	No change for 1/2 hr (2.3%)

[a]Incidence at Cleveland Metropolitan Hospital.
Modified from Sokol et al., with permission.

assess the problem and use clinical judgment to treat this patient based on the patient's needs. Possible interventions at this time could include (1) patience (do nothing), (2) ambulation, (3) augmentation with oxytocin, (4) use of analgesia, (5) regional block, or (6) membrane rupture. Vertex descent is not normally expected at this time.

EXAMPLE OF PROTRACTION IN THE ACTIVE PHASE (Figure 7.4)

A G3 P2 term patient with vertex in the LOP position was found to be 8 cm dilated at 1 pm. At 3 pm she was 9 cm dilated. The vertex position and station were unchanged.

Comment

This case fits the definition of a protraction of the active phase. At this point the clinician should consider intervention. Expect slower cervical dilatation when the vertex is in a posterior or transverse position, or with a poorly flexed head. The cervix may not retract as rapidly until further descent and rotation take place. Interventions include *no* intervention, that is, patience (a tincture of time is an acceptable intervention), or any of the measures noted in the previous example, including analgesia or oxytocin. Do not consider cesarean delivery on the basis of the protraction because this labor should continue. With an incompletely dilated cervix, forceps should not be considered.

EXAMPLE OF FAILURE TO PROGRESS

A 26-year-old G1 P0 has been in active labor for 10 hours and has reached 7 cm dilatation. For the next 2 hours she failed to dilate further. Based on several calls from the nurses, her physician made a diagnosis of failure to progress and began preparation for cesarean delivery. However, upon careful review of the patient's contraction pattern and a reevaluation of her pelvic capacity, it was decided to augment the labor with oxytocin first. After 30 minutes of augmentation, the patient became completely dilated and progressed to an uncomplicated vaginal delivery.

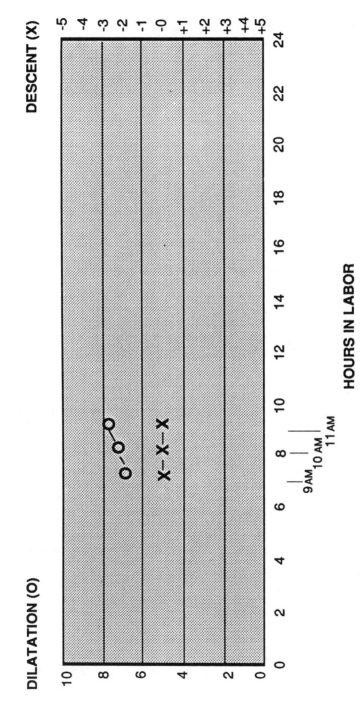

FIGURE 7.3

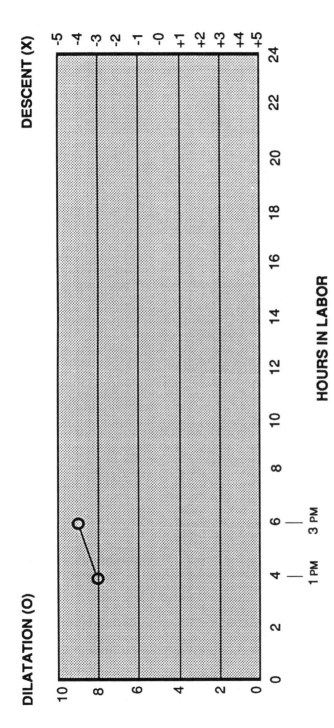

FIGURE 7.4

Comment

This case emphasizes that a patient must be carefully evaluated before operative delivery is undertaken. A careful evaluation of the patient's labor by the clinician is essential, even though there are subjective reports from others that it is adequate. In the situation in which the fetus is not stressed, attempts to improve the labor pattern should be undertaken. Likewise, reliance on the reports of others can result in unnecessary surgery.

Descent Phases of Active Labor

Because vertex descent may occur during active phase labor as well as the second stage, it is described here as well as in Chapter 8.

Onset

Vertex descent usually begins late in the active phase. In many labors, especially those of primigravidas, descent may not begin until the cervix is fully dilated. Descent may also occur later in the multipara but usually progresses with greater rapidity once it starts. In the nullipara, the vertex is usually at lower stations on admission, but descent occurs more slowly. If, after full dilatation between two vaginal examinations, 1 hour apart, descent has not begun, or having begun stops, either a protraction or an arrest is defined (Table 7.3).

Arrest

In contrast to cervical dilatation, the clinical decision that occurs in the management of vertex descent in the second stage of labor may be more difficult. Rarely should delivery be attempted through an incompletely dilated cervix. A high-forceps intervention should not be attempted in today's practice of obstetrics.

Factors Confounding Evaluation of Active-Phase Descent

Confusion in evaluating descent may be encountered because of caput formation and molding of the vertex. Both formation of caput and vertex molding will take place in the absence of descent, and in performing a vaginal examination the clinician must allow for these fetal changes when estimating change of station. The longer the labor, the easier it is to incorrectly estimate that greater descent has occurred when, in fact, only vertex molding and caput formation have taken place. Be conservative and, if in doubt, underestimate the pelvic station of the vertex.

Transverse and occiput posterior positions also confuse the estimation of descent. More molding and caput may form, and more time will be needed for descent to take place. In the occiput posterior position the vertex is usually poorly

Table 7.3 Abnormalities of Descent

	Nullipara	Multipara
Protraction	<1 cm dilatation change/hr	<2 cm dilatation change/hr
Arrest	No change in dilatation in an hour	No change in dilatation in 30 min

After Cohen and Friedman,[4] with permission.

flexed and the biparietal diameter is farther from the presenting part of the vertex. More errors may be made by the clinician inferring lower station than actually may exist. Over the years, the use of forceps in these situations has decreased, and this is to be encouraged. The choice of a difficult forceps after an abnormal second stage should be uncommon.

Four Factors Altering Progress in Active Phase

Parity

Station

Dilatation

Membranes

Clinical management is an art rather than a single pattern of care. Patient care must be individualized. Previous clinical experiences provide the basis for judgment and interventions.

In labor, evaluating the importance of many of the variables affecting cervical dilatation and vertex descent is difficult. The beginning clinician prefers a number to be given, or a line to be drawn, beyond which an action should be taken. (Rates for the length of labor are guides. The mother in labor requires individualized assessment.) There is, in fact, a great deal of latitude for patient care during labor. In the absence of fetal distress, there is no rush to complete the labor.

Parity and its Contribution to Labor Length

We expect nulliparas to progress differently than multiparas during labor. Nulliparas generally have longer latent phases and longer second stages. In contrast, during active phase the numbers 1.2 cm/hr and 1.5 cm/hr represent little measurable differences in cervical dilation rates and are difficult to perceive when attempting to estimate cervical dilation during a vaginal examination—a most imprecise measurement.

EXAMPLE OF THE LACK OF MEANING
OF THE PRECISE DILATATION RATE

Using the rate of cervical dilatation of 1.2 cm/hr for nulliparas and 1.5 cm/hr for multiparas, the majority of patients in the two groups will have rates of dilatation between 1 and 2 cm, and progress will appear to be the same throughout labor. It is only when hundreds of labors are averaged that the differences become apparent.

EXAMPLE OF THE LACK OF MEANING
OF THE PRECISE LENGTH OF ACTIVE LABOR

The length of active phase for the nulliparous patient group is 5 hours. The length of active phase for the multiparous group is 4 hours. Once again, the numerical differences are hardly of use. More often the length of the latent and second states correlate more closely with parity and parity contributes more to labor length.[3]

Vertex Station: A Need to Use the Same Measurements

In general, most clinicians use five stations above and below the ischial spines described by centimeter divisions (also an estimate) for the five pelvic stations (Table 7.4). On the other hand, some clinicians use three stations of the pelvis, which relate to finger breaths above and below the spine. For simplicity in understanding descriptions of labor, it is recommended that everyone use the five-station terminology, which more accurately reflects vertex station.

In Table 7.4, if the presenting part is palpated at or below the ischial spines, the widest part of the vertex presentation may be expected to be within the pelvic inlet. At that point it is appropriate to anticipate that vaginal birth should not be obstructed due to bony disproportion between the size of the vertex and the size of the pelvis. If the vertex is occiput posterior or occiput transverse, the distance between the fetal presenting part and the entrance of the fetal biparietal diameter into the inlet is longer. In this situation, although the head may feel engaged, the tip of the presenting part must be palpated at a lower station than 0, or the widest vertex diameter may still be above the inlet.

Consider also caput and molding of the vertex. These factors, when present, contribute to a more conservative estimate of the station of the vertex. It is safer to estimate a vertex higher than it feels on vaginal examination when molding or a large caput is present.

EXAMPLE OF PELVIC STATION AND PREDICTING LABOR LENGTH

A primigravida at station +3 (of five stations) still has significant time before crowning and birth. In contrast, S+3 (of three stations) suggests imminent delivery.

Table 7.4 Pelvic Stations

Three Pelvic Stations	Five Pelvic Stations	
–3	–5	Pelvic Inlet
–2	–4	
	–3	
–1	–2	
	–1	
0	0	Ischial spines (engagement)
1	1	
	2	
2	3	
	4	
3	5	On the perineum (vertex in view with contraction)

Comment

This may seem insignificant. However, a forceps is a midforceps at S + 3 of five stations, and a low or outlet forceps at S + 3 of three stations. In the courtroom this is useful information. It is time all concerned use the same definitions; five stations to define the pelvis should become standard. In Chapter 11 forceps will also be defined by pelvic station.

Vertex Station and its Contribution to Labor Length

In early labor the fetus of the nullipara is usually lower in the pelvis than the fetus of the multipara. On the other hand, in this same nullipara, descent to S + 5 (the perineum) may occur later in active or second stage and will be slower when compared with the descent in the multipara, in which descent, once started, moves rapidly. Station of the vertex at labor onset contributes little to the length of labor; that is, only 1% of the known reasons for length of labor are influenced by the station of the vertex in the pelvis[2] when the patient goes into labor.

It is important to place station of the vertex in proper perspective for clinical use. A high station for the nullipara or multipara may be associated with a longer labor, although station is not the major predictive factor of labor length. Similarly, a high pelvic station does not allow the clinician to predict labor failure prior to a trial of labor. In an extreme case, if the vertex is out of the pelvis, perhaps even overriding the symphysis pubis, the clinician should be looking for reasons for this fetal position. Is the patient obese? Is the placenta low lying or a placenta previa? Is the fetus of excessive size, or is the vertex abnormal in shape? Is a pelvic kidney present? (Pelvic kidneys may not always obstruct vertex descent.) In the absence of overt pathology with the presence of a high vertex, a labor trial is indicated.

Cervical Dilatation and Labor Length

In contrast to station and parity, dilation of the cervix contributes to the clinician's ability to predict how long the labor will be. About 4% of the known reasons for length of labor are derived from cervical dilatation.[2] However, in reality, this is not really very helpful as most reasons for labor length are not quantifiable. For example, one cannot quantify the effect of maternal contractions, position and flexion of the fetal vertex, or maternal relaxation or position during labor and predict how these variables will influence labor length. Many parts of labor are still not defined scientifically and have great degrees of variability from patient to patient. Estimating and judging are arts that improve with clinical experience.

Amniotic Membranes and Labor Length

Large patient populations and sophisticated statistical analysis are needed to document the very small (1%) known effect of artificial membrane rupture (AROM) on length of labor.[2] With this knowledge in mind, there should be no routine plan to rupture membranes for the individual patient. In some patients AROM will help speed up labor. In others it may hinder progress. In most cases artificial membrane rupture is of little help.

EXAMPLES OF DECIDING ON WHETHER TO RUPTURE THE MEMBRANES

At entry into the labor suite, a multipara was found to be a vertex presentation LOT, with a cervix 5 cm dilated and at station 0. The amniotic membranes were intact. How should the membranes be managed?

Comment

Some obstetricians routinely rupture membranes at this time. However, when there are no patient problems, there is little to be gained. Why rupture membranes now? If progress is good, there is no need to intervene. Membranes should not be ruptured to routinely visualize amniotic fluid or to insert internal fetal monitors in the absence of fetal or maternal problems. If fetal risk is suspected and the clinician wants to rule out meconium, individualize the clinical approach to the patient. If the external electronic monitor is not recording accurately and the information is important in a particular labor, rupture the membranes and apply an internal fetal monitor.

EXAMPLE OF USING MEMBRANE RUPTURE AS A TREATMENT FOR ARRESTED LABOR

A multipara with a normal size fetus was found to be arrested in active phase labor at 5 cm, S-1, vertex LOT, and with membranes intact. How should the membranes be managed?

Comment

One appropriate intervention is to perform AROM. Other possibilities should also be considered. Oxytocin stimulation would be appropriate. Information needed in this case is the quality of the uterine contractions and the amount of patient discomfort.

With all the information, there are several choices. Although AROM is not used in a routine fashion, when labor is not progressing it is a treatment of choice.

Other Variables That Affect Labor Length

Vertex position

Clinic pelvimetry

Cervical effacement

Fetal size

Labor environment

Vertex Position

The effects of posterior and transverse positions of the vertex, of flexion or extension, or even of vertex asynclitism (flexion to right or left) on the length of the active phase of labor is not well documented and is subject to much interpretation. In fact, the clinician rarely expects a posterior positioned vertex to descend rapidly through the pelvis. The nonanterior diameters are often less efficient delivery mechanisms and require more energy and time for pelvic muscles to stretch and the vertex to mold, flex, and rotate. When these positions are seen, expect a longer labor course.

Clinical Pelvimetry

Clinical pelvimetry is an important tool, although some clinicians continue to consider clinical mensuration useless. In this text clinical pelvimetry is presented and advocated for use in an attempt to deliver adequate patient care.

The shape of the maternal pelvis may be such that vertex rotation to an anterior position may not occur until the shape of the pelvis allows rotation to take place. Therefore, rotation may take place at a lower than anticipated pelvic station. In some labors, internal vertex rotation may even occur on the perineum. In other patients, the vertex will deliver from a posterior position without rotation. Pelvic shape also applies to fetal size considerations, for example, a platypelloid pelvis (characterized in part by a wide sacrosciatic notch) may accommodate a large head more easily in transverse positions.

Clinical pelvimetry should be initially performed at the first antepartum visit. It may be repeated during labor, but it is not as easily performed at that time. It should be noted also that each time a vaginal examination is performed during labor there may be temporary loss of some vertex station or dilatation.[5] This loss of station may depend on how vigorously the vertex and pelvis are examined, and clinical pelvimetry requires a more complete examination.

Cervical Effacement (and Position)

Another clinical variable that is difficult to quantitate is cervical effacement. In one examination an 80% cervical thickness measurement may be reported by examiner as an uneffaced cervix, while another examiner may indicate effacement is complete. Since the association with labor length and cervical effacement is based on clinical experience and statistics are not available, it becomes important to use general principles.

In general, the thinner the cervical effacement the more easily and rapidly dilatation will take place. Similarly, the posterior position of the cervix, in contrast to a midpositioned cervix, often foreshadows a longer labor course. Cervical position may be linked with vertex position. The occiput posterior or occiput transverse vertex positions are more common with the posterior cervix. No interventions are suggested. Cervical length or thickness may indicate that labor will be longer or shorter, but is still a speculation.

Membrane rupture should only be cautiously performed in the presence of a poorly effaced cervix. If the membranes are ruptured, will the presenting part descend and be apposed against the cervix? If following membrane rupture the vertex does not descend against the cervix, difficulty in continuing cervical dilatation may take place. In some cases there may actually be loss of dilatation or regression if membranes are ruptured. It is important to note that this discussion of membrane rupture refers to augmentation or treatment of labor. It doe not refer to initiation of labor.

Fetal Size

The larger fetus may be expected to progress through the pelvis more slowly than the average-size fetus. There is more vertex for the cervix to dilate and retract over, and there is more pelvic and vaginal musculature to be stretched. The smaller fetus with a smaller vertex has a shorter active and second stage of labor. Variable fetal size should be considered in management plans.

Some obstetricians suggest that excessive fetal size is defined as a fetus over 4500 g (9.9 lb) and when present it should lead to an elective cesarean in order to avoid shoulder dystocia.[7] It is true that shoulder dystocia occurs more frequently in large-sized infants; however, the majority of large-size fetuses deliver normally and without shoulder problems. In fact, the majority of cases of shoulder dystocia occur in normal size fetuses.[7] If labor is continued in the presence of a large fetus, it is appropriate to be less aggressive in management. For example, in a patient with a large fetus and failure to descend to the perineum, the use of midforcep may be associated with shoulder dystocia.

The Patient Care Environment

It is difficult to assess the effect of the patient care environment on the length of active-phase labor. In general, patients relate to good environmental support, improved comfort, removal of anxiety, and the facilitation of relaxation. All of these effects may shorten labor, but how much the environment affects labor is a speculation. The sounds coming from some labor rooms today appear to be symphonies of fetal heart beats. Is this good or does this detract? If a noisy patient is in labor, does this have an impact on other patients? These are all unanswered questions.

EXAMPLE OF THE EFFECT OF ENVIRONMENT ON LABOR

A patient in early latent-phase labor was observed and monitored for 20 hours. She arrived at 1 cm dilatation and progressed to 6 cm dilated with vertex S–2. She was tolerating labor poorly. There was a protraction of the active phase during the previous 2 hours, when she progressed from 5 to 6 cm.

Comment

Any healthy person lying in bed for 20 hours, relatively restricted in movement and always hearing the fetal heart monitor, should be exhausted. This mother needs help. Choices include medication for rest or a regional block. This situation inevitably makes labor tolerance by the mother and management by the physician more difficult. Perhaps the best cure for this patient would have been to remain home for a longer pert of her latent phase.

Active-Phase Interventions

The importance of the labor diagnosis is reemphasized. If progress is continuous and at 1 cm or more per hour, there is usually no need to intervene. If protraction or arrests are present, potential interventions include:

1. Patience
2. Ambulation/position change
3. Medication/analgesia
4. Regional anesthesia
5. Oxytocin
6. Cesarean

In the absence of fetal distress, there is no reason to effect a surgical end to labor without first trying to make a diagnosis. Why is the labor problem happening?

Treat the problem. In some cases it is appropriate to end labor prior to an adequate labor trial. On the other hand, many interventions have the potential to increase infant or maternal morbidity. There is a great amount of latitude within the treatments available.

Risk for infant neurologic injury following abnormal labor patterns was analyzed at Cleveland Metropolitan General Hospital.[8] The abnormalities, defined by protractions and arrests in active labor, and interventions such as oxytocin use, did not correlate with neurologic morbidity in infants 2 years after birth. Neither vaginal nor cesarean birth routes demonstrated improved clinical outcomes or altered neurologic damage.

The active phase of labor is the portion of labor in which most obstetrical clinical management skills are called upon. In one management situation, the cesarean may be appropriate and will terminate the labor without continuing the physician's anxieties, which are generated in caring for a patient when labor is not proceeding well. In contrast, management of a nonsurgical nature takes more time, occurs in an environment of increasing patient and physician discomfort, and raises fetal risk questions that are ill defined. For example, it is not known how long active-phase labor may persist, or how much molding or pressure on the fetal vertex can be sustained during second-stage labor without increasing the risk for fetal morbidity.

The neglected and prolonged labors of the past were traumatic to the mother and fetus. As a guide, a prolonged labor may be defined as a labor that extends more than two standard deviations from an arithmetic mean of all labors. The numbers are not synonymous with brain damage. No study has shown that a 3-hour second-stage labor is more morbid than a 2-hour second-stage labor.

In this section two previously described concepts are reintroduced: orderly *diagnostic evaluation* of the clinical problem, and *therapeutic intervention* for treatment of the laboring patient. The goal is to be sure that all interventions are considered before failure of vaginal birth occurs.

Management of Active-Phase Labor Abnormalities

Transition Phase

The transition time from latent to active phase is depicted in Figure 7.5 at A. It is inconstant in time and simply a change in the rate of dilation from slow to more rapid.

1. When in doubt, treat as if in active labor.
2. When at 5 cm, treat as active labor.
3. Note the shaded block in Figure 7.5 at A may occur earlier than 3 cm or later than 5 cm of dilatation.

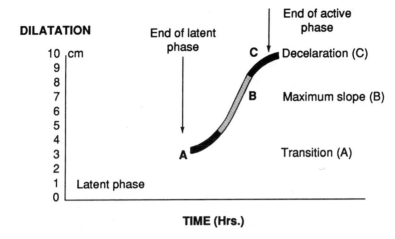

FIGURE 7.5

Maximum Rate of Dilation (Figure 7.5 at B)

The area described as the maximum rate of dilatation is seen in Figure 7.5 at B (dotted line). At this point in labor, since there is a good indication as to how fast a cervix will dilate by comparing the dilatation examinations of the patient, the clinician may anticipate the length of the labor.

Format for Analyzing and Treating Abnormalities

Chart notes, as discussed for latent-phase labor, should include a description of the patient's history (if this is the first note rather than a progress note) and management plans. Active-phase diagnosis and treatments are introduced again as terms, not to suggest some new methods for patient care, but rather as part of an orderly process. Document what has occurred. Think of what may be done. Consider all patient care options and intervene. This process should be described in the chart note.

Describe the labor. A note is usually made at the first patient contact during labor. Thus, if the patient has already been admitted and examined, begin at point number 4 below.

1. Include a brief statement about relevant maternal or fetal background factors, including general medical history and the antepartum course. This should be the first note in the admitting obstetrical record.

2. Is the patient in active labor? After two examinations there should be a note in the patient's chart describing her progress and answering this question.

3. List the intrapartal clinical factors that are important, including cervical dilatation, station, and vertex position.

4. Conclude with a brief description of labor thus far. The interval note is written in the patient's chart. In contrast to latent-phase labor, when it may not have been possible to describe the observed labor course, in active-phase labor there is a labor course to review. The orderly documenting of this information helps to clarify the clinician's thinking during the long hours of labor. Years later the note may be helpful for review purposes.

Examples of Active-Phase Labor Abnormalities

The chart notes should be similar to the notes describing the diagnostic evaluation in cases of active phase labor abnormalities. In the examples, the therapeutic sequences, when possible, are presented as flow diagrams with two possible outcomes. Judgment for a therapeutic intervention in these examples may differ among individual physicians evaluating the same case. Several interventions may be acceptable. Clinical care involves judgment; the evaluation is subjective, altered by recent experience and often differing when comparisons between clinicians are made. The different physician responses to the same clinical experience suggest that there are usually several options for patient care.

EXAMPLE OF DIAGNOSIS AND TREATMENT OF PROTRACTION AND ARREST OF CERVICAL DILATATION (Figure 7.6)

A 28-year-old nullipara with a normal antepartum history stated that her contractions began 4 hours prior to admission. She was observed in the hospital between 2 and 5 pm with progress from 5 to 6 cm of cervix dilation, 80% effaced, and with the vertex OA at station −3. Her membranes were intact. A 3700-g fetus was estimated. The maternal history was unremarkable. The patient stated that she had not slept well for the past 2 days and was extremely tired. It was apparent she was not tolerating her contractions well. The electronic monitor displayed contractions, each 3 to 4 minutes, with normal heart rate information.

Diagnosis Chart Note

This previously normal patient has a protraction of the active phase as documented by slow dilatation of cervix (1 cm in 3 hours). Although contractions have been moderate, little progress has been made.

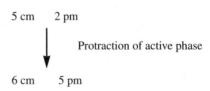

5 cm   2 pm

Protraction of active phase

6 cm   5 pm

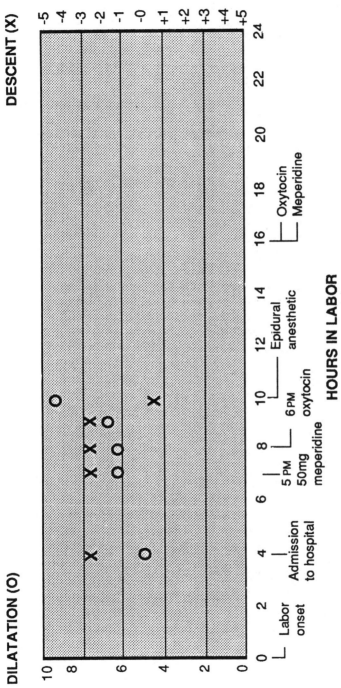

FIGURE 7.6

Therapeutic Choices

1. *Patience:* Waiting longer is probably not a good idea without other support (medication for pain or rest).

2. *Ambulation:* This choice is similar to the patience option. The patient will not walk easily in her present tired, anxious, and painful state.

3. *Medications:* Meperidine is acceptable. About 50 mg intravenously in a normal-size patient is used.

4. *Regional block:* Epidural anesthesia may also be helpful. However, because the uterine forces may be part of the problem, also consider oxytocin augmentation of labor.

5. *Stimulation (oxytocin):* As noted in point 4, oxytocin use is highest on the list of choices to be used in conjunction with some form of pain relief. Medication in a tired patient may lead to 3 to 4 hours of rest with little progress unless oxytocin is also used. At other times, pain relief may rapidly increase labor progress.

6. *Membranes:* Many obstetricians would perform artificial rupture of membranes (AROM) as a treatment to improve labor. If oxytocin were used, even more clinicians would rupture the membranes to facilitate internal electronic monitoring. If it is believed that the vertex will not be well applied to the cervix after AROM, membrane rupture should be delayed. In addition, it is not mandatory to perform internal monitoring when using oxytocin if the external monitoring data are acceptable in quality, but it is mandatory to monitor. The information must be technically readable.

7. *Mechanical (forceps/vacuum):* This is not an acceptable intervention at this time.

8. *Cesarean:* This is not an acceptable intervention at this time.

The Labor Continues

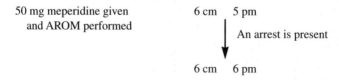

50 mg meperidine given
and AROM performed

6 cm   5 pm

An arrest is present

6 cm   6 pm

New interventions should be considered because there was no change. The arrest of labor in active phase warrants further treatment.

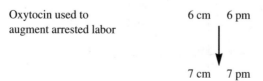

Oxytocin used to
augment arrested labor

6 cm   6 pm

7 cm   7 pm

Comment

In the absence of progress, consider problems such as fetal size or position (perhaps the examination of vertex OA position was incorrect). This patient is proceeding in labor like an OP. However, since some progress has occurred (from 6 to 7 cm) the plan is to keep the patient comfortable and to continue treatment.

Oxytocin continues   7 cm   7 pm
Epidural added for pain relief

9 cm   8 pm
station   0

Comment

The patient is near the end of the active phase. A decelerative phase may follow. The new progress appears acceptable. Patience is now added to the clinical routine. As long as progress continues and no indicators of fetal distress are observed, this slow labor, despite the fact that abnormalities (protraction and arrest) have been present, will end in a vaginal birth.

The therapeutic interventions in this case have been

1. Patience
2. Medication (meperidine, epidural)
3. Stimulation

EXAMPLE OF EARLY INTERVENTION IN QUESTIONABLE LABOR (Figure 7.7)

A 39-year-old G3 P2 mother at 41 weeks of gestation has had a normal antepartum history. Labor contractions began 4 hours ago. On admission to the hospital at 1 am, the patient was noted to have a term-sized fetus, with intact membranes, vertex OP at –3, cervix 3 cm dilated, 80% effaced, with painful contractions every 7 to 12 minutes.

Diagnostic Chart Note

In the presence of a normal antenatal history there is no unusual fetal risk. It is uncertain as to whether the patient is in the latent phase of labor. However, because the patient is at term and the cervix appears to be inducible, an induction will be attempted in order to observe the fetal and maternal responses. The membranes will not be ruptured unless there is an indication for this.

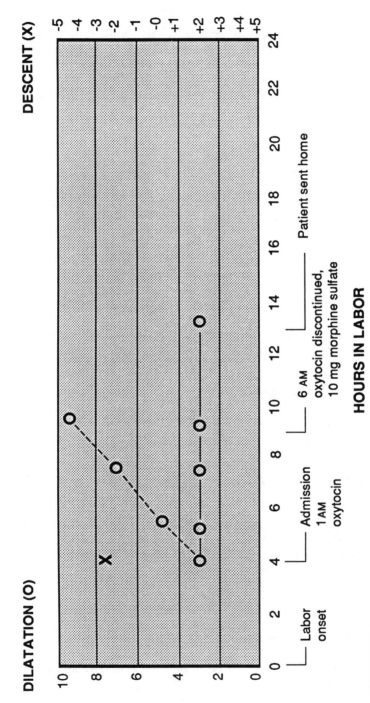

FIGURE 7.7

Comment

Maternal age at term in a healthy mother adds no fetal risk during labor. In the office, and without contractions, many clinicians might consider an induction or would suggest that the patient remain at home. In the labor room, in the presence of painful contractions, many clinicians would modify that approach. Despite the factual statement about no increased risk at age 39, inevitably the clinician is influenced by this fact. At 41 weeks of gestation and with an inducible cervix, induction of labor at the next convenient time (i.e., early the next day) warrants consideration.

Therapeutic Choices

1. *Patience:* This is a possibility and acceptable; other obstetricians may choose to intervene more aggressively.

2. *Ambulation:* Same as point 1.

3. *Medication:* This is a possibility. However, the patient did not appear tired. Rarely use Seconal in the presence of pain. Meperidine analgesia may be considered for this patient. In general, try to avoid medication early in labor or until labor is well established. Occasionally use medication for pain relief or anxiety at any stage of labor.

4. *Regional block:* Epidural analgesia would not be considered this early, unless the patient's reaction to pain was extremely unusual.

5. *Oxytocin:* In this case, the clinician chose to stimulate the patient. However, the obstetrician did not commit herself irrevocably to complete the labor as the membranes were not ruptured. If oxytocin therapy did not result in cervical dilatation, the clinician could turn off the oxytocin and even send the patient home.

6. *Membranes:* Many clinicians would choose to rupture membranes at the time of induction. Some benefit is gained from looking for meconium in the amniotic fluid. Try not to rupture membranes unless there are reasons to persist with the induction. If problems in the technique of monitoring arise or fetal distress is questioned, rupture the membranes, insert a pressure catheter, and attach a scalp lead.

7. *Forceps/vacuum:* This is not considered at this time.

8. *Cesarean:* This is not considered at this time.

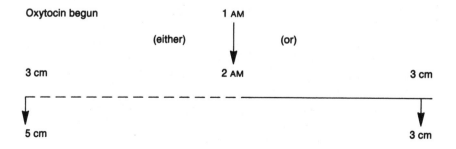

If the cervix had dilated to 5 cm the induction would have been continued.

If the cervix had remained 3 cm dilated, continuing the induction for several additional hours would be considered (Figure 9.3).

If the cervix becomes fully dilated, the patient is managed as a normal labor, and vaginal delivery is anticipated in the next several hours.

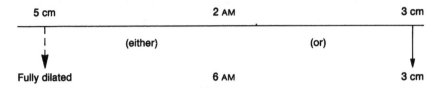

In the alternate situation, with no progress at 3 cm, in the absence of fetal heart-rate abnormalities, stop the oxytocin, medicate, and rest the patient, or even send the patient home after the effects of oxytocin have stopped. This decision is predicated on the condition of the patient, including her fatigue, contractions, stress, and personal desires.

History

At 3 cm oxytocin was discontinued and the patient was rested with 10 mg morphine for 4 hours. She awoke with an unchanged cervix and irregular contractions.

Intervention

There is still choice. If induction is started now, look for a long labor. Consider sending the patient home, see her in 2 to 3 days, check the cervix, and await labor. The fetal heart monitoring was reassuring.

Fetal Distress During Active or Second-Stage Labor

Up to this point active-phase labor problems have been considered in the absence of fetal distress. The diagnosis of fetal distress all too frequently appears as a secondary diagnosis when decisions for interventions such as cesareans are made. In reviewing charts of cases such as these, linkage of the diagnoses "failure to progress in labor and fetal distress" occurs too frequently to be acceptable. It appears that the heart-rate monitor may provide too easy an excuse to complete the labor. A "little dystocia" and a "possibility of fetal distress" are considered equivalent to a single correct diagnosis of either dystocia or fetal distress. To be prudent, always consider the possibility of abnormal labor producing fetal distress. The increased frequency of "failure to progress in labor" and "possible fetal distress" leading to a cesarean cannot be explained.[18]

If fetal distress is suspected because of a change in fetal heart beat-to-beat variability, or the observation of occasional variable decelerations (which are common in many labors and are not generally risk factors), obtain better information. Fetal scalp blood examinations are not always helpful. Between 1975 and 1984, one of the two major reasons for the yearly increase in cesarean birthrates was the increased use of the diagnosis of fetal distress.[5] It is unlikely that obstetricians have learned better methods for identifying fetal distress. Fetal concerns cannot be ignored. In a difficult labor close attention must be paid to all labor events. The diagnosis of dystocia and fetal distress are defined. They should be used accurately when intervention takes place during a difficult labor.

Summary

1. Active-phase labor has three parts:
   a. Accelerative phase
   b. Maximum slope of dilatation
   c. Decelerative phase
2. In the active phase, the rate of cervical dilation should equal or exceed 1.2 cm/hr for the nullipara and 1.5 cm/hr for the multipara.
3. Vertex descent usually takes place late in the active phase or during the second stage of labor.
4. Arrests of descent include no change for 1 hour in the nullipara and no change for 1/2 hour in the multipara.
5. Active-phase labor pathology or poor progress is not indicative of fetal damage.
6. Mean rates of labor do not infer morbidity by themselves; they are guidelines to alert the clinician to intervene.
7. Timely chart notes should document the patient's labor course and the clinician's outcome expectations.
8. In the chart note, all therapeutic interventions and the reasons for continuing, adding, or changing the patient care plan should be listed.
9. Friedman graphs should be plotted in the chart as the patient is being examined during labor.
10. Active-phase interventions include:
    a. Patience
    b. Ambulation
    c. Sedation, analgesia
    d. Regional block
    e. AROM
    f. Oxytocin
    g. Cesarean

11. Forceps use should be reserved for second-stage interventions.

12. In the absence of obvious maternal or fetal risk factors, there will often be several clinical choices. Management choices will differ among clinicians, even when considering the same case. There are few absolutes in clinical care.

References

1. Shiono PH, McNellis D, Rhoads GG. Reasons for the rising cesarean delivery rates. Obstet Gynecol 1987;69:696–700.

2. Peisner DB, Rosen MG. The latent phase of labor in normal patients: A reassessment. Obstet Gynecol 1985;66:644–648.

3. O'Driscoll K, Meagher D. Active Management of Labour. London, WB Saunders, 1980, p 106.

4. Cohen WA, Friedman ER. Management of Labor. Baltimore, MD, University Park Press, 1983, Chapter 2.

5. Sokol RJ, Nussbaum RS, Chik L, Rosen MG. Computer diagnosis of labor progression V. Reliability of a subroutine for evaluating station and descent of the fetal presenting part during labor. J Reprod Med 1974;13:183–186.

6. Acker DB, Sachs BP, Friedman EA. Risk factors for shoulder dystocia. Obstet Gynecol 1985;66:762–768.

7. Bottoms SF, Sokol RJ, Rosen MG. Short arrest of dilatation: A risk for maternal and fetal infant morbidity. Am J Obstet Gynecol 1981;140:108–116.

8. Rosen MG, Debanne SM, Thompson K. Arrest disorders and infant brain damage. Obstet Gynecol 1989;74:321–324.

9. Sokol RJ, Stoikof J, Chik L, Rosen MG. Normal and abnormal labor progress. I. A quantitative assessment and survey of the literature. J Reprod Med 1977;18:47–53.

Chapter 8

Second Stage of Labor

Overview

In Chapter 7, active-phase labor was characterized in terms of medical management. As a surgical procedure, the cesarean was considered only after medical management had been tried and failed. In marked contrast, historically, the second stage of labor has involved a large surgical component. Although most fetuses deliver spontaneously, second-stage labor interventions include the use of forceps, the vacuum extractor, and the cesarean. It is in the second stage of labor that physical trauma to the mother and fetus may take place. The second stage of labor is a time when both the patient and clinician may be physically and emotionally exhausted, and when interventions to end labor are expected.

The second stage of labor begins with full cervical dilatation and ends with fetal birth. The interventions for second-stage labor have important historical precedents that presage today's rationale for clinical care.

Objectives

At the conclusion of this chapter, the clinician should be able to

1. Define the second stage of labor
2. Understand the historical precedents for various interventions
3. Determine appropriate medical and surgical interventions for the second stage of labor
4. Define the pathologies consequent to second-stage labor interventions

Evolution of Second-Stage Labor Management

In one of the more famous obstetrical stories, Sir Eardley Holland, as quoted by Hellman and Prystowsky,[1] described the death of Princess Charlotte following what was obviously an arrest in labor. Sir Richard Croft, the princess' physician, was faced with the dilemma of intervening to save the life of Princess Charlotte and destroying the fetus (the future king of England), or performing a cesarean to save the fetus, most probably leading to the death of the princess (the future queen of England). Neither treatment forecast a satisfactory outcome, and, in the dilemma created by the two choices, Sir Richard chose to do nothing. Ultimately, both members of the royal family, princess and future king, died. Sir Richard committed suicide sometime later, perhaps in remorse over this tragic outcome.

The introduction of the use of forceps gave obstetricians an alternative to the cesarean, which, at that time, inevitably led to the mother's death. Appropriate forceps use became an obstetrical debate more than 100 years ago and still continues today. Soon after their introduction, forceps use became the hallmark of the obstetrician, which separated him from the midwife. In contrast, today midforceps use in second-stage labor carries with it an almost unspoken stigma and is rapidly becoming lost as an obstetrical skill. Neither extreme appears appropriate.

In 1820 Merriman (again quoted by Hellman and Prystowsky[1]) wrote, "Forceps shall never be applied until the ear of the child has been within reach of the operator's fingers for at least 6 hours." Thus the 6-hour rule was introduced. Other rules were soon to follow. Even today clinicians often quote and act according to a 2-hour rule, the origin of which Hellman and Prystowsky also describe.[1] Most clinicians practicing today accept the fact that should be considered the second stage should be no longer than 2 hours or it is abnormal and should be ended. Shortening of the second stage of labor to the 2-hour rule was brought about by Delee.[1] He urged the application of "prophylactic forceps" in a paper read before the American Gynecological Society in 1920.[1]

The medical value of the 2-hour rule was studied for morbidity by Hellman and Prystowsky[1] at the Johns Hopkins Hospital between 1937 and 1949. During that interval prophylactic forceps were used to shorten the second stage of labor. About 3% of all labors exceeded a 3-hour second stage, with a median second-stage duration for multiparas of 20 minutes, and 50 minutes for primiparas. The authors observed that prolongation of the second stage was associated with increased postpartum hemorrhage, puerperal infection, and infant morbidity. This classic paper also foreshadowed Friedman's later studies of labor and delivery. The authors noted an association between first-stage labor abnormalities and second-stage problems, and also observed the effect of posterior vertex positions on labor length.[1]

Evaluation of the link between labor abnormalities and fetal and neonatal morbidity continued in more current studies by Bottoms et al.,[2] although this retrospective review did not distinguish whether fetal complications were already present and produced neonatal morbidity, or whether the labor abnormalities produced the wastage. It was clear that significant differences in neonatal neurologic morbidity were not found when both occurred either by the cesarean or vaginal route following protractions or arrest. Wayne Cohen,[3] studying the lengths of second-stage labors, found no increase in depressed Apgar scores or neonatal morbidity in second stages prolonged beyond 3 hours. He did notice that there was infection, as Hellman and Prystowsky had noted many years earlier. It is notable that the Bottoms report was followed by a long-term study by Rosen and Debanne that confirmed the neonatal study.[4] This report came from an obstetrical service where midforceps use was rare, and may reflect the separation of a prolonged second stage of labor from a difficult forceps birth. The confounding variables of prolonged second-stage labor, or fetal distress, cannot easily be separated from the effects of midforceps applications when attempting to determine later neurologic risk for the infant. This area of dystocia and forceps is reviewed again in Chapter 11. Thus, although we define second-stage labor as onset with full dilatation, and there are mean values to describe average lengths, an arbitrary rule by number, such as the 2-hour rule, is not acceptable as a concept to end labor.[5]

Definition of Second-Stage Labor (Table 8.1)

Classic descriptors may be used for the definition of the second stage of labor. Second stage labor begins at full cervical dilatation and ends with the birth of the neonate. If there is pathology in the second stage of labor, the vertex does not descend (failed descent), descent progresses too slowly (protraction of descent), or descent stops after starting (arrest of descent).

The use of time limits and rules are guidelines for interventions. Morbidity cannot be predicted either in long or short second-stage labor. If, as one would logically believe, there is some point beyond which the second stage of labor becomes morbid, that length of time is not known to the clinician. The 2-hour rule appears arbitrary and often too short. A 3- or 4-hour rule cannot be made without data. In fact, many clinicians do follow patients in second-stage labor for 3 and 4 hours in the presence of normal fetal monitoring of term infants and when descent is slow but continuing.[5]

Character of Normal Descent During Second-Stage Labor

Descent is progressive and usually begins later in the active phase. More multiparas are unengaged at labor onset and may stay that way until the second stage is well underway. Cephalopelvic disproportion associated with a mismatch of fetus with pelvis size cannot be accurately assessed until the patient is well into the active or second stage of labor.

The nullipara usually enters labor at a lower pelvic station, but descent may not begin until the second stage is established. While it is taught that most nulliparas will demonstrate vertex engagement at labor onset, that dictum more correctly refers to the patients perceived signs of "lightening" and the abdominal examination conducted with Leopold's maneuvers, which may confirm that the vertex is

Table 8.1   Second-Stage Labor Definitions

Failed	No descent is noted from time patient is first examined
Protraction (in second stage)	Nullipara: Descent <1 cm/hr
	Multipara: Descent <2 cm/hr
Arrest (in second stage)	No change *after* descent has begun
	Nullipara: 1 hr
	Multipara: 30 min

Modified from Friedman and Sachtleben,[1] with permission.

relatively well placed within the pelvis. On vaginal examination it is often found that the presenting part is still above the ischial spines. Further vaginal descent will begin to take place after labor onset, but often not until the decelerative portion of the active phase or the second stage of labor.

The second stage of labor tests pelvic capacity for fetal size. In most patients, irrespective of pelvic size, the cervix will continue to dilate around the fetal head, even though descent does not take place. The diagnosis of cephalo-pelvic dispro-portion cannot be made with accuracy until full or almost full cervical dilatation has been reached. Perhaps in a very small number of patients, clinical pelvimetry can predict absolute disproportion; however, few patients have that small or dis-torted a pelvis so that the clinician may say the fetus will not deliver vaginally.

Factors Associated with Abnormalities of Second-Stage Labors

Active-phase labor abnormalities show consistent associations with problems in the second stage of labor. This is in contrast to latent-phase abnormalities, which do not predict labor problems.[6] Protractions and arrests in the active phase may be associated with descent problems.[7] If active-phase labor abnormalities have already been noted, the clinician should anticipate second-stage abnormalities.

Maternal and Fetal Size, and Clinical Pelvimetry

Maternal size, particularly for the very short patient (under 5 ft tall), is a consid-eration. But even in the short mother, clinical estimates are rarely indications to prevent a trial of labor. Maternal size, along with clinical pelvimetry, estimates alert the clinician to a potential for labor problems, which allows for earlier inter-vention than in a labor where there appear to be no factors suggesting pelvic dis-proportion. Excessive maternal weight (with respect to height) should also be listed as a risk factor.

Fetal size over 4000 or 4500 g may be useful in raising suspicion that second-stage labor may be prolonged. Size may be a concern; yet, the majority of large fetuses deliver normally. Thus the clinical impression is only additional informa-tion to be processed and used in the management plan. Increased fetal size is associated with increased maternal prepregnancy weight and also with excessive weight gain during pregnancy. Therefore, in the presence of these maternal risk factors, carefully document fetal size.

The clinical maternal and fetal size risk factors provide guides that caution the clinician to avoid aggressive interventions. Some of these conditions include: a large fetus, a diabetic mother, or a preexisting active-phase abnormality. The clinician may consider medical interventions (time, analgesia, oxytocin), but good judgment dictates earlier termination in the management of these labors. It would be of value to supplement the clinician's examination with ultrasonographic evidence of fetal size near term.

Clinical Interventions in Second-Stage Labor

Possible interventions of second-stage labor include:

1. Patience
2. Ambulation
3. Stimulation (oxytocin)
4. Analgesia
5. Regional anesthesia
6. Cesarean
7. Forceps/vacuum

The decrease in the use of all forceps during the last 25 years has been appropriate. Labor should be completed without excessive force. A difficult labor, terminated by the use of difficult forceps, is associated with increased risk for fetal and maternal trauma.

EXAMPLE OF MORE TIME GIVEN FOR THE SECOND STAGE
(Figure 8.1)

A normal nullipara at term with an estimated 7-lb fetus has been in labor for 12 hours and has been fully dilated for 1 hour. The vertex is LOT. During the last 3 hours the vertex has progressed from station –1 to station 0.

Comment

This is not an uncommon clinical finding during the second stage. By definition, this is a protraction of descent. However, in the OT position anticipate slower descent as vertex flexion, molding, and then vertex rotation must take place. Watchful waiting is appropriate as

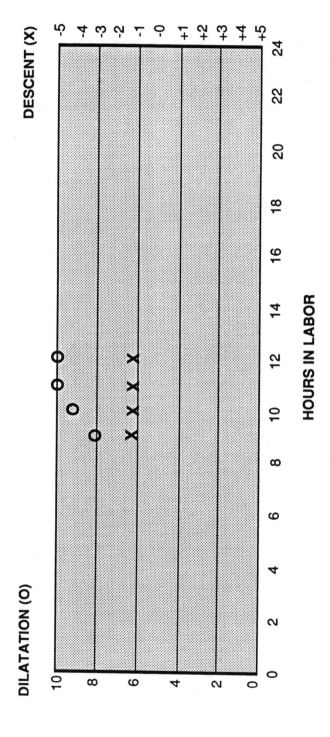

FIGURE 8.1

long as progress continues. An arbitrary 2-hour rule is not acceptable. An alternative plan for this patient could include ambulation. During ambulation monitor the fetal heart each 5 minutes with auscultation or a Doptone device. The use of oxytocin is acceptable if it is felt that the contractions are not as strong as they should be. The use of analgesia or anesthesia is appropriate if maternal pain or poor relaxation is a consideration. Forceps intervention or a cesarean are not considered at this time. The vertex may be engaged despite the molded vertex, which is felt at the ischial spines.

Anesthesia or Analgesia

Pain relief with the use of regional anesthesia, such as the epidural, will provide relaxation of pelvic muscles. Some clinicians argue that epidural anesthesia increases the use of forceps, and that descent and vertex rotations may not take place as easily. The question has not been resolved. When there is the need for pain relief or failure to rotate or descend is present, regional anesthesia is another therapeutic choice. If failure to rotate or descend follows an earlier regional block, it can be overcome with oxytocin stimulation, or by allowing the anesthetic to "wear off."

It is impossible to predict the effect of pain-relief therapy. The clinician has this option for treatment, which is reversible and incurs little risk. Rapid cervical dilatation and vertex descent may follow medication use. Rapid dilatation and descent have also slowed following this same intervention. Thus, the medication use should not be routine; it should be used selectively and for pain. On the other hand, pain relief should not be denied when indicated.[8]

Oxytocin

Bell-shaped contractions may be apparent on the fetal monitoring tracing, yet the expected cervical dilatation and vertex descent may not take place. Even if palpation indicates adequate contractions at the bedside, cervical dilatation and descent may not take place. The final guide for patient care is the rate of cervical dilation in active-phase labor and vertex descent in second-stage labor. If, after starting oxytocin, descent does not take place in a progressive manner, disproportion must be considered and new interventions are indicated.[9]

EXAMPLE OF OXYTOCIN SUPPLEMENT FOR FAILURE TO DESCEND DURING THE SECOND STAGE (Figure 8.2)

In a multipara, following 8 hours of progressive labor, epidural anesthesia was administered at full cervical dilatation and the vertex at station –2 in the LOT position. During the next

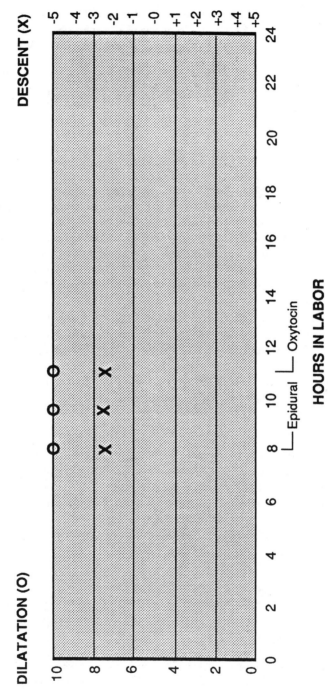

FIGURE 8.2

2 hours the vertex failed to descend. The fetal heart-rate tracing continued to display normal findings. Because the fear of recurrence of the labor pain was an important consideration for this patient, rather than discontinuing the analgesia the obstetrician used oxytocin stimulation.

Comment

Oxytocin use was appropriate in this case and is appropriate in the presence of protractions or arrests of descent. Continuing observation must take place when these "next steps" are considered. In this case, although contractions appeared adequate, no progress was being made. Judgment involves watching the fetal heart rate to be certain that the addition of oxytocin does not lead to deprivation of supply to the fetus, as may be demonstrated by periodic delayed decelerations or diminished heart-rate beat-to-beat variability. Frequency of contractions and adequate return to normal pressure baselines between contractions is reassuring. However, prolonged use of oxytocin without progress is to be discouraged.

The clinician should always consider using oxytocin in the presence of what would appear to be good uterine contractions. Contraction shape or perceived intensity is not satisfactory unless progress is made. In this situation, following the use of oxytocin expect progressive descent in 1 hour. If no progress continues and no monitoring abnormalities are present, oxytocin use may continue. Be cautious before considering any forceps as an intervention in difficult second stages of labor. Try to avoid the midforceps as an intervention. At a point when descent has been a second-stage labor problem, move to cesarean rather than midforceps, even if the head has become engaged. After 3 or more hours in second-stage labor, the vertex, with its molding and caput, is probably not as low in the pelvis as it may appear. Avoid what may be anticipated difficult midforceps.

EXAMPLE OF A LONG SECOND STAGE AND OXYTOCIN USE FOLLOWED BY PROGRESS (Figure 8.3)

After 10 hours of labor, a P2 G3 mother was fully dilated and at station +1 for 2 hours. The vertex was OA. An arrest of descent was diagnosed at station +1. The monitoring tracing displayed uterine contractions every 3 to 4 minutes, with occasional coupling of contractions. Oxytocin stimulation was instituted. The vertex descended during the next hour to station +2.

Comment

Although the second stage was 3 hours in length, progress was taking place. In the absence of electronic fetal monitoring abnormalities, continued stimulation was reasonable. Midforceps use for slow progress at this time would be inappropriate. Avoid getting involved in the sequence of an arrest followed by oxytocin use with some progress, and then followed by midforceps application. As noted earlier, there is no guide to determine how long to continue the labor before giving up on the vaginal birth. The decision as to when a cesarean should be performed must be individualized. If progress continues, the decision may be made to allow more time in labor. If progress stops while using oxytocin, or if progress does not take place, cesarean birth is the choice. There are no hourly rules. The 2-hour rule is too

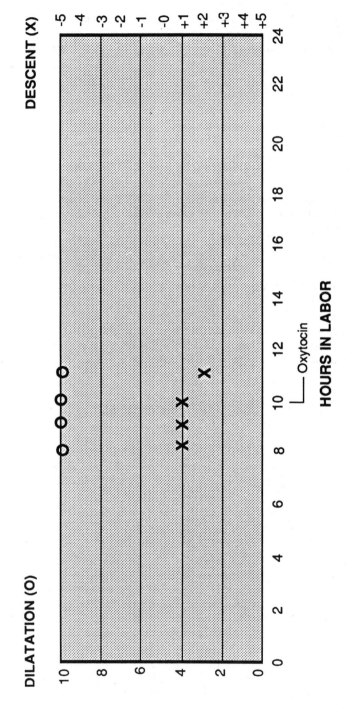

FIGURE 8.3

arbitrary. Judgment is needed. In contrast to the term infant, in the presence of fetal distress or a low-birthweight fetus, interventions would be more rapid.

EXAMPLE OF AN ARREST OF DESCENT AND THE 2-HOUR RULE (Figure 8.4)

After a 14-hour labor, a P0 G1 mother with vertex OP was at station +2 and fully dilated. No change in station had taken place for 2 hours. She was stimulated with oxytocin. During the next 2 hours vaginal examinations confirmed increasing caput and molding. Although it appeared that descent was occurring on vaginal examination, the obstetrician, allowing for the change in the size and shape of the vertex, felt descent was minimal or absent, and chose to perform a cesarean rather than to persist.

Comment

In the absence of fetal emergencies, do not use forceps between station 0 and +2 in a five-station pelvis. Try other measures, such as time, regional anesthesia, or the use of oxytocin, although failure to observe progress with oxytocin use leaves few options. The length of time observation may be continued is uncertain. Most clinicians stop oxytocin use in active or second-stage labor in the absence of observed progress after 1 or at most 2 hours of a trial. This clinical situation, with the vertex engaged, takes place relatively infrequently. Usually, the vertex arrests at higher stations. When the fetus is in the pelvis at this level, expect continuing descent to take place. However, in posterior positions much more vertex molding takes place and that takes time. Despite the patient being haltered with a monitor and oxytocin in the venous lines, maternal position may be changed, and the patient may even be ambulated. If ambulation is used, monitoring (telemetry, if available, or Doptone) must continue. If oxytocin is being used, monitoring should be continuous. Another intervention to be considered in low-station-descent arrests is epidural anesthesia along with oxytocin augmentation. Pelvic relaxation may facilitate vertex descent.

Forceps/Vacuum Extraction

Forceps and vacuum extraction are additional therapeutic interventions for use in the second stage of labor. Forceps use should be defined and classified by station. A complete discussion of forceps use is covered in Chapter 11.

EXAMPLE OF FORCEPS USE TO SHORTEN SECOND-STAGE LABOR

A nulliparous mother was exhausted following a 20-hour labor. The vertex was at station +5 in OA position. The vertex was seen on the perineum without spreading the labia with each contraction. The mother could not push out the fetus. A low forceps was effected for maternal indications.

124

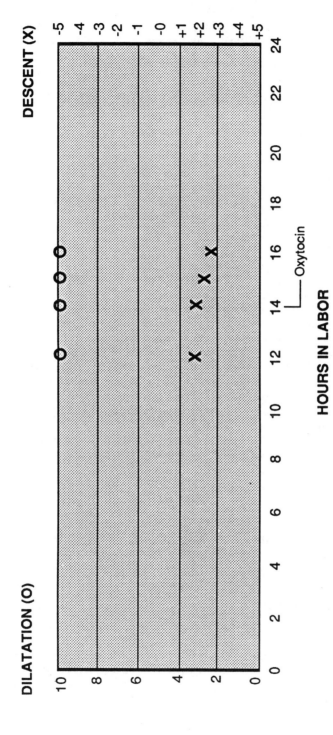

FIGURE 8.4

Comment

The use of forceps or vacuum from low station to shorten the second stage is acceptable if the mother's situation calls for their use. Some clinicians would describe this as an outlet forceps and confine the definition for low forceps to station +4. As noted in Chapter 11, classifying forceps by station and rotation adds more information and removes the categories low, mid, and outlet forceps, which have varying definitions to obstetricians.

EXAMPLE OF MATERNAL EXHAUSTION IN A VERTEX OCCIPUT POSTERIOR (VOP) POSITION

A nulliparous mother had been actively "pushing" during the second stage of labor for the past 2 hours. Inspection of the perineum revealed dilatation of the vagina with each contraction, but the vertex could not actually be seen by the examiner without further labial separation. The vaginal examination revealed molding and caput with the vertex as station +4, and in an LOP position.

Comment

The reason the vagina separated and yet the vertex was not visualized without spreading the labia was that in the OP or OT positions, wider diameters of the vertex separate the vaginal walls before crowning is seen. Allowing more time would be effective. If the patient is taken to the delivery room at this point without crowning taking place, the forceps birth will be more difficult than expected. Although, because of the molding, the vertex feels lower in station, this vertex is more likely at station +2 or +3. The vertex is deliverable, but it will require more traction force. By definition, this is a midforceps delivery if the station is +4 or higher. Alone with other medical interventions, use of regional anesthesia, such as epidural blockage, may facilitate vertex descent while preserving the ability to "push."

Station +2/+3

A vertex at station +2 to +3 (of five pelvic stations) should be expected to deliver vaginally. This may not always occur spontaneously. If a second-stage descent abnormality follows regional block during a normal labor, several therapeutic choices are available (time, oxytocin, or allowing the medication to wear off). In the absence of fetal distress, forceps use and the cesarean should be deferred. In fact, it may be difficult to deliver a station +3 vertex by cesarean because of the depth of the vertex in the pelvis.

Stations +2 and +3 contrast with lower pelvic stations (remember, in this text five stations to the pelvis are used); therapeutic interventions are always more worrisome at this point of labor. Following a protraction of the active phase or in association with an arrest of descent, the decision to use forceps should be most cautious. With skills that should be acquired during resident education, vaginal birth in most cases can be effected with forceps. However, once a protraction or arrest of descent has taken place, be wary of forceps use. They will usually be more difficult and may presage a larger fetus or difficulty with the shoulders.

EXAMPLE OF ACTIVE AND SECOND-STAGE LABOR ABNORMALITIES (Figure 8.5)

A multiparous patient had a latent phase of 12 hours. During active-phase labor she arrested for 3 hours, at station –2 and 7 cm cervical dilatation. The fetus was normal in size and the contractions appeared adequate. The patient was exhausted. She was given 50 mg of meperidine intravenously. At the same time, augmentation of labor with oxytocin resulted in slow progress. Three hours after oxytocin use, the patient was fully dilated and at station +2. This situation is thus a long active phase with slow progress. Two hours later dilatation was at station +3.

Comment

In this case, beware of the use of midforceps. The cesarean is a prudent decision. This has been a difficult labor with active and second-stage pathology. Despite what the clinician may think he or she feels, allowing for caput and molding, the vertex is probably not at station +3. In most examples such as this, once oxytocin has begun, consider also the use of regional anesthesia to provide muscle relaxation and pain relief.

It is important to have neurologic data relating to midforceps use as assessed by each station of the pelvis. Friedman's data derived from the Collaborative Cerebral Palsy Study in the 1960s and Dierker and Rosen's data from the Cleveland Metropolitan General Hospital in the 1970s suggest different conclusions about forceps use and will be discussed. Midforceps use in the presence of protractions or arrests is not easily advocated. Even if the operator believes he or she is skillful enough to effect vaginal delivery, caution is advised as a protraction or arrest in the second stage may foreshadow more difficulty in the delivery.

Use of Fetal Monitoring with Active and Second-Stage Abnormalities

The patient without antepartum risk whose labor progresses normally need not be electronically monitored if the fetal heart rate can be auscultated each 30 minutes during the latent phase and each 15 minutes during the active phase. If labor progression during the active and second stage does not occur at the expected rate and intervention is considered, electronic monitoring should be instituted. When oxytocin is used, both external and internal monitoring modes are acceptable. These cautionary measures regarding monitoring are taken with the understanding of both the benefits and limitations of monitoring.[10]

For example, it is accepted that too frequent contractions from oxytocin use may be associated with delayed decelerations or fetal bradycardia. The visually

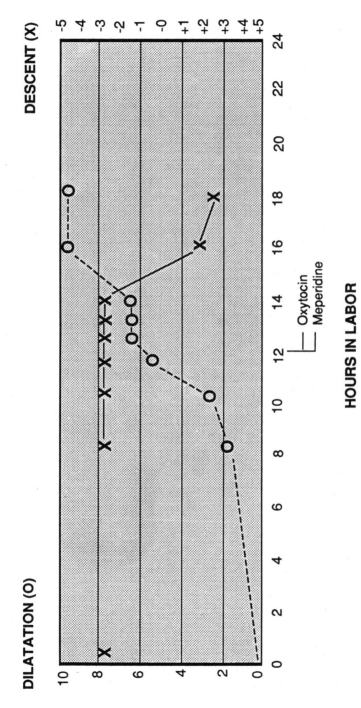

FIGURE 8.5

displayed patterns allow for quicker diagnosis and treatment. However, the absence of fetal heart-rate abnormalities, for example, in the presence of an arrest of labor in the active phase, or an arrest of descent during the second stage of labor, does not always portray intracerebral events secondary to the difficult labor that may foreshawdow cerebral injury. Thus, the clinician must rely on prudent judgment in treating the problems. Stated differently, we do not have information that allows for rules to be set on the length of time one should allow for labor or the use of oxytocin. One cannot depend on electronic fetal monitoring for these answers.

Throughout this book references have been made to the too frequent use of the cesarean during the latent and active phases of labor. An adequate trial of labor in order to test pelvic capacity has been the major theme. However, cesareans performed during the second stage of labor are not usually criticized. Time for allowing the vertex to mold, flex, rotate, and descend is continuously stressed. The second stage is not the heart of the cesarean debate. One clinician may choose to perform a cesarean in the presence of an arrest of descent at station +3 based on training and recent clinical experience. Another clinician may choose forceps based on different training. The high cesarean birthrate is less associated with the use of the cesarean during the second stage of labor. If an adequate trial of labor has been given, the cesarean avoids Sir Richard's dilemma of not intervening.

Strict adherence to the 2-hour rule is not valid and must be replaced by clinical judgment. The absence of observed fetal distress suggests that neuropathology does not follow unless a traumatic delivery takes place, but the monitor is limited in this area. Stated conversely, more time allowed for delivery without forceps does not appear to be traumatic.

Summary

1. The second stage of labor begins with full dilatation and ends with birth.

2. Descent of the vertex usually begins late during the active phase of labor and continues through the second stage of labor.

3. Pathologies of second-stage labor include:

    Arrest of descent (no progress): >1 hr nullipara
    >30 min multipara
    Protraction of descent: <1 cm/hr nullipara
    <2 cm/hr multipara
    Failed descent: No descent during labor

4. Treatment interventions for second stage include:

    a. Patience

    b. Ambulation

    c. Analgesia and anesthesia

    d. Stimulation

    e. Low forceps, midforceps, vacuum extraction

    f. Cesarean

5. Second-stage pathologies are associated with delay or failure of the vertex to rotate, descend, or flex well. Fetuses in these positions often do not conform to the expected labor patterns.

6. Compared with other stages of labor, it is in the second stage of labor that pelvic capacity is tested.

7. Clinical judgment involved in choosing when and how to terminate second-stage labors is difficult to define and may be considered the "art" of patient care. The relationship between neurologic morbidity, abnormal labor, and birth route choice is still being debated.

8. Arbitrary termination of second-stage labor at the end of 2 hours is inappropriate when slow progress in descent continues.

9. Following abnormal second-stage labors, the midforceps should be used infrequently and with caution.

References

1. Hellman L, Prystowsky H. The duration of the second stage of labor. Am J Gynecol 1952;63:1223–1233.

2. Bottoms SF, Hirsh JJ, Sokol RJ. Medical management of arrest disorders of labor. A current overview. Am J Obstet Gynecol 1989;156:935–939.

3. Cohen W. The influence of the duration of the second stage labor on perinatal outcome and puerperal morbidity. Obstet Gynecol 1977;49:266–269.

4. Rosen MG, Debanne SM, Thompson K. Arrest disorders and infant brain damage. Obstet Gynecol 1989;74:321–324.

5. Menticoglou SM, Manning F, Harman C, Morrison I, Perinatal outcome in relation to second stage duration. Am J Obstet Gynecol 1995;173:906–912.

6. Peisner DB, Rosen MG. The latent phase of labor a reassessment. Obstet Gynecol 1985;66:644–649.

7. Friedman EM, Sachtleben MR. Station of the presentation: Pan V. Protracted descent patterns. Obstet Gynecol 1970;36:558–567.

8. ACOG. Pain Relief During Labor. Committee opinion #118, 1993. Washington, DC, American College of Obstetricians and Gynecologists.

9. ACOG. Dystocia and the Augmentation of Labor. Technical bulletin #218, 1995. Washington, DC, American College of Obstetricians and Gynecologists.

10. ACOG. Fetal Heart Rate Patterns: Monitoring, Interpretation and Management. Technical bulletin #207, 1995. Washington, DC, American College of Obstetricians and Gynecologists.

Chapter 9

Dystocia
The Pathology of Labor

Overview

Previous chapters have reviewed the organization of patient care, described neurologic morbidity with respect to labor, defined terminology for the labor stages, and presented treatment programs for abnormal labor patterns. In general, all terms and definitions conform to the Friedman nomenclature, which allows for better communication. The use of well-defined terms allows the clinician to intervene in a more orderly and prompt manner when labor is not progressive. In this chapter on the pathology of labor, which is very broadly defined, dystocia is presented as a concept to be placed in the dictionary of terms.

The terms *dystocia* and/or *failure to progress* are frequently used in obstetrical diagnoses. They are reviewed in an attempt to remove them from the readers' glossary of terms. These terms are vague and have different meanings to different investigators. Words such as *cephalo-pelvic disproportion* (CPD) have a definite meaning but are often misused or poorly understood.

Howard Taylor, writing in the foreword of Moloy's monograph[1] on pelvic measurements, stated that "cephalopelvic disproportion is the chief cause of difficult labor, and difficult labor is still the most important problem in obstetrics." Although many years have elapsed since that statement was made, it is still correct today. The term *cephalo-pelvic disproportion,* with all of its descriptive vagaries, encompasses a treatment problem responsible for about one third of the primary cesareans performed in the United States.[2] It is difficult to believe that in an era of less crippling illnesses such as poliomyelitis, less bony pelvic distortion due to rickets or scurvy, improved treatment of trauma, and better nutrition, the female pelvis appears less adequate to accommodate vaginal delivery. Yet, the use of this term as a diagnosis made by obstetricians continues to be a major treatment problem.[2,3]

Objectives

At the conclusion of this chapter, the clinician should be able to

1. Understand the meaning of *dystocia* and replacement terminology with respect to success in vaginal birth
2. Accept the Friedman classification as an adjunct to patient care
3. Describe abnormalities of labor in a chart note in terminology that will allow peer review of labor progress
4. Describe in detail the clinical situation rather than use terms such as *failure to progress, dystocia,* and *cephalo-pelvic disproportion* in chart notes as indicators for treatment

Brain Damage

The diagnosis of a difficult labor should be described in terms of protractions or arrests in the active phase, and in the second stage, or as arrests of descent of the vertex. These diagnoses are always made retrospectively, after labor difficulty has become evident, and the fetus had already experienced a portion of labor. The obstetrician is not clairvoyant and should rarely use a labor diagnosis to justify terminating labor in the latent phase or before labor onset.

There are data since the mid-1970s that conclude alteration in birth route as a treatment for abnormalities of labor does not alter the incidence of brain damage.[4,5] Note that this more recent evaluation is not the description perceived as a neglected labor nor as a traumatic delivery, which was commonly seen in the patient care of previous eras. Today, while the sun may rise on a single labor, it rarely rises twice on a woman in labor.

In a review by Bottoms et al.[4] from Cleveland Metropolitan General Hospital, dystocia, defined by protractions and arrests, was not associated with evidence of neurologic morbidity during the neonatal period. The same infant population was reviewed in a follow-up after 2 years of age, or when major neurologic morbidity was first documented.[5] Obstetrical treatments, such as the use of oxytocin, forceps, or cesareans, which were used as interventions in these difficult labors, were studied for their relationship to major brain damage.

The use of oxytocin was not associated with increased infant brain damage when compared with neonates born after similar problem labors which delivered without oxytocin.[5] In this particular patient care environment, oxytocin use was carefully controlled. Cesareans were rarely performed before a trial of oxytocin was instituted. The usual practice was to start oxytocin and then to anticipate progress within 1 hour, and usually to desist within 3 hours in the absence of progress, during active-phase or second-stage labor. In the Cleveland study, whether delivered by cesarean, low forceps, or midforceps, infant neurologic outcome remained the same. Forceps use in the population was uncommon.

It cannot be stated that any abnormality of labor is harmless, because the study did not compare them with normal labors. Prospectively, there is no way to avoid an abnormality before it occurs. The available treatment regimens described here are acceptable on the basis of known infant outcome.

In summary, brain damage is not changed by changing birth route in patients. The variate here is that good judgment is applied in labor management. Intervene if progress does not take place as expected. Heroics or difficult forceps after difficult labors are not acceptable.

Repeat Cesareans

Evidence of the inability of clinicians to define what dystocia really is may be found in studies of vaginal birth after a cesarean for dystocia. More than half of the patients who have had a trial of labor following a cesarean for a diagnosis of dystocia delivered vaginally, and with larger neonates.[6] Some of the responsibility for the outcome of the primary cesarean for dystocia must rest with the obstetrician's judgment of allowing, or not allowing, for an adequate trial of labor. Some difference in outcomes in the following pregnancy may also include better fetal adaptation to the maternal pelvis. Fetal size apparently is not the problem. Understanding the outcome of labor and birth with respect to clinical pelvimetry and fetal size, mechanical forces of labor, and behavioral influences affecting labor is at best an inexact science. A diagnosis of dystocia as an indication for a previous cesarean should not exclude a trial of labor in the following pregnancy.

Criteria for Definitions

As noted in Table 9.1 in the past innumerable terms have been used to describe labor. In this text labor is described in terms of latent, active, and second stages, and the Friedman criteria, with minimal modifications, are used. If clinicians use a uniform language and similar definitions, such as those listed in Table 9.2, outcomes between different obstetricians acting on different risk patients with different patterns of care may be compared and evaluated. This will lead to more consistent guidelines for labor management.

Etiologies for Abnormal Labors

No matter how the clinician tries to determine specific etiologies for abnormal labors, there is a tendency to speak in vague general terms using clinical "feelings" and traditionally worded descriptions. For example, in the most specific of circumstances, with a catheter documenting intrauterine pressure during a contraction, a cervix may not dilate and it will not be known why dilation did not take place. The catheter may document symmetrical contractions with adequate pressure peaks, but if the cervix does not dilate, the labor will not progress despite the normal pictures. For these reasons, our treatments of labor protractions or arrests

Table 9.1 Inappropriate Terms for Describing
Abnormal Labor

Dystocia
Cephalopelvic disproportion
Failure to progress in labor
Pelvic contracture
Excessive size fetus

---

are at best pragmatic, involving a series of intervention trials and successes or failures. As long as the principles applied to the various treatments involve avoidance of increased risk to the mother and fetus, it is appropriate to continue the labor.

Abnormalities of women in labor have been described in terms of (1) problems of the birth canal; (2) problems of fetal position, presentation, and size; and (3) problems of the forces of labor. Assessment of these three general categories requires assessment of the two patients involved. A vaginal examination, ultrasonography, or viewing contractions portrayed by an electronic monitor, when used alone is inadequate clinical care. Taken in the context of the entire patient picture, tests and evaluations are helpful, but they can only be used to assist the clinician in reaching a diagnosis.

Assessing the Mother

Maternal Stature

The female pelvis is only part of the patient's complete physical picture. Maternal height may have an association with pelvic size. The very short or disproportionately built patient may foreshadow problems during labor because of pelvic size. However, for the individual patient, the predictive value of the data about maternal height are vague at best.

The very obese patient may have problems of soft-tissue dystocia. These women do have a higher incidence of larger babies.[7] Despite the risks, most obese patients deliver large babies at term without difficulty. Maternal stature alerts the clinician to suspect a potential for a problem, but at best the actual risk for the problem will be quite small. Similarly, the vaginal birth risks may be balanced against maternal anesthetic risk and postoperative morbidity, all of which are increased in association with cesarean birth.

Measurements of the Birth Canal

Clinical measurements of the pelvis have already been described in Chapter 3. They are best performed early in pregnancy before the fetal vertex is in the pelvis. During labor, because of fetal position, poor pelvic muscle relaxation, or maternal *able 9.2* Labor Diagnosis[a]

erm	Criteria[b]
Prolonged latent phase	Nulliparas >20 hr
	Multiperas >14 hr
Protracted active-phase dilatation	Nulliparas <1.2 cm/hr
	Multiparas <1.5 cm/hr
Arrest of dilatation	No progress for 2 hr
Protracted descent	Nulliparas <1 cm/hr
	Multiparas <2 cm/hr
Arrest of descent	No progress for > 1 h

[a]Modified from Friedman's criteria.
[b]Numbers indicate 95th percentile.

discomfort, pelvic measurements may be difficult to perform. As an example, most pelvic sidewalls feel convergent when examined during labor.

The following three measurements may be helpful during labor:

1. The *diagonal conjugate* is too short if less than 11.5 cm, and may foreshadow a problem labor in which the vertex may not engage. This measurement is less easily made during labor, because it is painful to perform and the vertex may be in the way.

2. The *prominence of the ischial spines* may help document the size of the midpelvis. If the vertex is at or near the ischial spines, the inlet usually has been traversed, the vertex is engaged, and thus a size mismatch between pelvis and fetal head should not be a problem. In contrast, prominent ischial spines may foreshadow problems in vertex rotation and descent in the midpelvis. Even in the presence of suspected prominent ischial spines and a short diagonal conjugate, dilation of the cervix should take place. The cervix should dilate, even if descent cannot be completed. The labor will declare itself if given adequate time. If the vertex does not descend it may not be applied to the cervix, and once again dilatation may become a problem.

3. The sacroscratic notch may also be an adjunct in determining the capacity of the midpelvis. If the distance from the ischial spine to the sacrum is less than 3.5 cm, it can mean a decreased capacity for the head to rotate. If this is combined with a deep sacral curvature, a posterior position of the occiput will commonly occur. On the other hand, if the sacral curve is absent or nearly absent, a transverse occiput will have difficulty rotating either direction.

This simplified description of intrapartum pelvic assessment does not infer that the shape, position, and curve of the sacrum; the size of the sacrosciatic notch (2 to 5 cm); and the splay of the side walls of the pelvis (convergent, straight, or divergent) are not all helpful. It is just that during labor these measurements are difficult to perform. As observed in teaching exercises with residents, or by the questions asked at residency and specialty examinations, it is apparent that there is a widespread lack of knowledge of pelvic architecture and of the measurements of the pelvis.

Some clinicians argue that attempting to measure or assess the clinical pelvis is a waste of time. In this text it is still presented as useful information. First, picture the three-dimensional shape of the birth canal; this assists in thinking in terms of why a vertex does not rotate or descend. There is a distance that must be traversed and adapted to for the passage to take place.

EXAMPLE

Some vertex presentations deliver the occiput posterior because of fetal size and maternal pelvic shape. The occiput posterior birth of an average-size baby will demonstrate a long molded vertex, far different from the occiput anterior vertex birth. This "shaping" of the head had to take place or the fetal diameters would not allow adaptation and descent to take place.

Knowledge of pelvic shape allows the clinician to think about birth mechanisms in terms of fetal and pelvic sizes and shapes. The pelvis as a birth canal becomes more easily visible.

EXAMPLE

If forceps are to be applied, the clinician should understand that there is a curve to the sacrum along which the pelvic curve of the forceps blade must be guided. Similarly, ischial spines impinge on the passageway and the forceps application must be guided by these points. In the presence of prominent ischial spines, if rotation is to be performed it should take place above or below the spines that are preventing spontaneous vertex rotation.

The vertex must flex and descend beneath the symphysis pubis before the vertex can be extended over the perineum. Lack of understanding as to where to flex the vertex under the symphysis may lead to increased pressure on the vertex. Early vertex extension leads to the use of more traction force and potential trauma.

Pelvis and Forceps Traction

When applying traction, understanding the three-dimensional qualities of the birth canal allows application of traction in a lower direction (towards the floor) when the vertex is above the perineum, and in a more horizontal direction as the vertex first flexes below the symphysis pubis and then extends after the occiput has passed under the symphysis. The use of pelvimetry provides a clinical concept of how birth may take place and how forceps traction may be used. This is discussed more thoroughly in the chapter on forceps.

Use of X-ray Pelvimetry and Tomography Prior to or During Labor

X-ray pelvimetry is no longer a useful routine and is not a required measurement for vertex births. In the preface to his monograph on pelvimetry, Thomas[8] noted that all patients on the University Service of the Grace New Haven Hospital during the previous 25 years had undergone x-ray measurements. That day is long since gone. Today, use of x-ray pelvimetry is infrequent. No recent studies documenting the usefulness of x-ray pelvimetry have been performed.

The evaluation of computed tomography is also ill defined. The technique may hold more promise for precise pelvic measurements. Before computer-averaged tomography (CAT) pelvimetry is accepted as useful, studies must be performed in a controlled manner demonstrating the prognostic accuracy of the technique. Also, with the active laboring patient or during the evening, night, and weekend hours, it is difficult to arrange a CAT scan.

Despite the above statements, all too often the radiologic demonstration of a below-average-size pelvis (still normal, not contracted, but just below average) is equated with too small a pelvis and is used as a reason for terminating labor (or avoiding it in the first place). A small pelvis is frequently diagnosed in the presence of breech presentation. The reported findings may represent an obstetrical bias against the vaginal delivery.

Assessing the Fetus: Fetal Size, Fetal Abnormalities

Fetal bony abnormalities, such as hydrocephalus or abnormal growths or tumors, speak for themselves. However, fetal size, large or small, is not usually an indicator for avoiding labor. Arguments have been made for arbitrarily setting limits for vaginal birth at 4500 g. No clear endpoint is available. Rather, the passenger and the pelvis need to be assessed.

In the presence of a large fetus, be wary of labors that do not progress easily and without stimulation. A vertex not engaged at labor onset is a usual finding with a large-size fetus. However, a greater concern is that in labor a large vertex followed by larger shoulders will engage the vertex, but when the vertex then delivers the shoulders will impact. On the other hand, shoulder dystocia is not predictable. While shoulder dystocia has a higher incidence with large fetuses, the majority of shoulder problems take place in normal-size fetuses. In general, when ultrasonography data predict the birth of a larger than 4000-g fetus,[9] the incidence of shoulder dystocia will rise. This should not be an excuse to avoid a trial of labor; however, this information should caution the clinician to limit interventions such as oxytocin or forceps. The delivery of the 4000-g fetus vaginally is acceptable and usual. There are more concerns about disproportion between fetal vertex and shoulders when estimates of fetal weight exceed 4500 g. Arbitrary fetal size limits are not suggested.

EXAMPLE

A large mother with a history of having delivered fetuses between 4000 and 4500 g is evaluated differently than an expected large fetus in a short, nulliparous mother.

Comment

There is no rule or standard beyond which size estimates of the vertex should be delivered by cesarean. Certainly in the 4000- to 4500-g range, caution and preparation for the birth is in order. Anticipating a large fetus, the obstetrician should prepare for the birth in a delivery room environment and with anesthetic support available, rather than in a birthing environment where emergency support will be limited.

Ultrasonography to Determine Fetal Size

With the use of ultrasonography, the documentation of fetal weight and size is quite helpful. It must be understood that at the extremes of fetal size there is less accuracy in the estimations. As noted in the preceding section, the use of a cesarean in fetuses between 9 lb (4000 g) and 10 lb (4500 g) is not mandated. Certainly more aggressive intervention, such as oxytocin or forceps use, should be considered with extreme caution. If the labor is proceeding well, allow it to proceed. If progress is poor or arrested, the labor-ending decisions are reached more easily. For the rare patient with an expected fetal weight beyond 10 lb, or 4500 g, look for antecedent medical problems, such as diabetes or maternal obesity. The clinician who uses a cesarean without a trial of labor in the 4500-g fetus has not infrequently found that clinical and ultrasonographic predictions of fetal size did not correlate with the neonatal weight. Many times the fetus estimated to weigh over 4500 g results in a 4100-g neonate. In general, await labor onset; then a judgment, which may vary between clinicians, is made. If the vertex descends and labor is proceeding well, deliver the patient vaginally. In contrast, with a high vertex at labor onset and slow progress, move promptly to a cesarean.

Fetal Mechanics

The way a fetus is moved through the pelvis during labor is poorly understood and rarely even considered. Labor necessitates adaptation of the fetal body and head to the maternal pelvis. The teaching of labor mechanics, for example, that in the vertex presentation there is internal rotation, descent, and flexion, and with birth there is vertex extension and external rotation, is a neglected part of clinical care education.

It may be helpful for the clinician to think in terms of the following patterns. If the vertex is in the occiput posterior or transverse position, it is generally poorly flexed. The vertex may be deflected or even extended. The fetus will need to descend and to flex in order to present a smaller diameter for birth, and labor will take more time.

An extended vertex may deliver vaginally if it extends or rotates. A face may deliver vaginally if it engages and rotates to a mentum anterior position. Many face presentations will remain high and will not engage. For example, if the vertex is extended and does not descend, think of a possible brow presentation, which is usually undeliverable vaginally.

When the cervix stops dilating in the active phase, look for an abnormality in fetal mechanics as well as uterine forces. Frequently, the cervix will not dilate completely if the vertex remains high and is unengaged in the pelvis. Rotation to an anterior position may not occur. In contrast, at the level of station +3 within the pelvis, the vertex in posterior position may deliver in that position. Because the occiput posterior diameters are larger than the occiput anterior diameters, far more effort is needed in this fetal situation and increased vertex molding and longer second-stage labors are anticipated.

Similar to problems of flexion and rotation, keep in mind lateral flexion or asynclitism (flexion to the side). These fetal mechanical problems create labor difficulties involving more pressure, more molding, and more time.

Problems that relate to the mechanics of labor generally do not occur in a single fetal diameter. Generally, vertex left occiput transverse also has asynclitism. These situations lead to more difficult labors associated with protractions and arrests of dilatation and descent. The Friedman system allows documentation of the problem but does not give the reasons for the problems. Treatment individualized to the clinical problem may include position change, ambulation, oxytocin, regional anesthesia, or combinations of these therapeutic measures.

Molding of the Vertex

It is not easily explained why some patients still in latent-phase labor and at high pelvic stations present with caput and molding of the vertex. At times, even overriding of the parietal bones at the sagittal suture may be seen with a vertex at relatively high stations of the pelvis. In contrast, some patients with relatively short latent and active phases, and with a fully dilated cervix, show little caput or molding of the vertex. The unmolded fetal vertex may need more time in the second stage of labor to acquire the molding before the vertex will deliver. Generally both caput and molding correlate with fetal size and labor length.

In today's' less aggressive vaginal birth environment, the occurrence of a dural sinus laceration secondary to excessive vertex molding, following a too long labor or a difficult forceps, should be rare. Cohen's data[10] on second stage labor show that in the second stage, time and patience beyond the 1- and 2-hour limits is acceptable. Thus, 3 or perhaps 4 hours of watchful waiting in the absence of fetal distress and in the presence of continuing progress is acceptable. Judgment and caution are also included in this plan. When descent is slow but continues, and the second stage lengthens, observation of continuing descent over time is appropriate. Intervention with midforceps should be infrequent because these labors foreshadow difficult instrument deliveries.

Assessing the Uterine Forces

Correlating Contractions with Progress

A protraction or an arrest of labor may be seen either in the presence of less frequent or less strong uterine contractions, or both. In a protraction or arrest of labor, one expects to see an analog of this pattern on the electronic monitoring record. In contrast, protractions or arrests may also occur, even in the presence of good contractions, that appear as bell-shaped curves associated with adequate intrauterine pressure levels and contractions each occurring every 2 to 3 minutes. This is not what is expected. The monitoring pictures and the patient's progress is good, but the monitor is not displaying the expected patterns. Similarly, stimulate a labor that is not progressing but in which the in-utero pressure pattern is as perfect as the expected contraction picture.

EXAMPLE

Contractions began 4 hours prior to admission in a G3 P2 at-term patient with normal antepartum and past history. She was admitted at 5 cm dilatation, vertex at station –2, 80% cervical effacement, and spontaneous rupture of membranes about 1 hour before admission (Fig. 9.1). An average-size fetus was expected. In the hospital during the next 2 hours, despite the presence of apparently adequate contractions, no progress was seen. Dilatation remained at 4 cm.

The obstetrician chose to medicate the patient with 50 mg of demerol intravenously and begin an oxytocin infusion. One hour later the patient was 8 cm dilated. At this time, an epidural block was administered for pain relief.

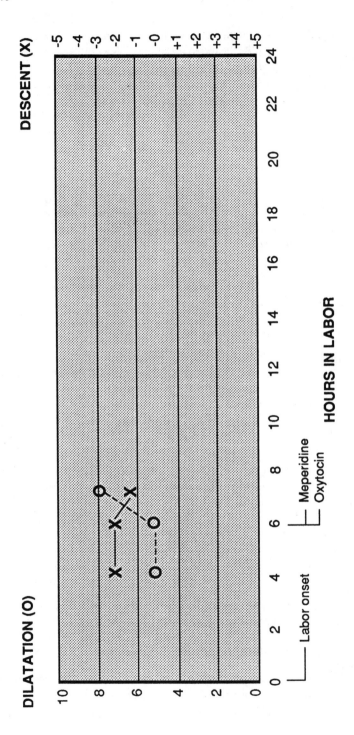

FIGURE 9.1

Comment

Many intervention choices were acceptable here. At 5 cm the patient is considered — if in labor — to be active phase. Without progress for 2 hours it is possible this was not labor but highly unlikely. The use of oxytocin was acceptable as long as monitoring confirmed an absence of fetal placental supply problems. Medication for pain relief was another Almost all treatment modalities except labor termination were acceptable in this patient alone, or in concert with the oxytocin.

Physiology or Pathophysiology of Contractions and Labor

Transition from the laboratory to the labor bed and from muscle contraction to labor understanding has been slow. It is not understood why labor contractions start and why labor begins. More is known about why and how the uterine smooth muscle contracts. Contractions can be stimulated or stopped. Yet little is known about the propagation of the contraction throughout the uterus and why electronic monitoring of some contractions produces a skewed curve displayed on the paper tracing and other contractions produce bell-shaped curves on the recording charts. Little is understood about the contraction pattern or its physiology. It is not understood why the contractions, good or poor, may or may not dilate the cervix. It is almost impossible to assess uterine forces or effectiveness of function accurately between the extremes of no contractions and tetanic contractions. For these reasons the clinician learns to judge labor not upon contractions but on cervical dilatation.

Criteria for Effective Contractions

The criteria for evaluation of uterine forces is a judgment made at the bedside and in association with clinical progress. Questions to be asked are as follows: Is progress, as documented by cervical dilatation, taking place? Is there a prolongation of the latent phase or a protraction or an arrest present in active or second stage of labor? This information is more meaningful than the shape and frequency of the contraction.

There are fetal questions to be asked in the presence of contraction abnormalities. Is the fetal heart rate recording normal? Specifically, is the tracing without evidence of late decelerations, which may indicate uterine flow is being restricted secondary to abnormal contractions? In summary, the criterion for effective contractions is good progress in labor associated with expected cervical dilatation in the absence of signs of fetal distress.

Dysfunctional Labor

Terms such as *dyscoordinate* or *dysfunctional labor* are frequently used and poorly understood. These terms do not adequately define the pathology of the problem and are not useful. The visual picture of frequent contractions with little progress in cervical dilatation is well known. In the presence of abnormalities of contraction frequency and shape, think in terms of the entire system — labor progress and fetal condition.

When the electronic findings suggest adequate forces are present but the clinical findings show poor progress, the choice of clinical interventions is not clear. Proceed in a trial and observation mode. In these situations consider ambulation in a rested patient and regional block before oxytocin use. However, even in the presence of what appears to be good uterine contractions, careful use of oxytocin may provide a more adequate trial of labor. Close observation and avoidance of any evidence of delayed decelerations or signs of fetal deprivation of supply or distress are needed.

Treatment Program for Abnormal Labor: Active Management Protocol

The active management system proposed by some authors involves graphing labor beginning from the time of entry into the labor suite and early intervention with oxytocin.[11,12] These authors are proponents of a system that does not define latent and active phases of labor. Labor is pictured as a straight line and is expected to progress with 1 cm/hr of cervical dilatation. Labor, which is generally defined by entry into the labor room, is completed in 10 hours. The second stage ends in 2 hours, usually without forceps and is associated with low cesarean birthrates. These authors[11,12] suggest that uterine rupture resulting from oxytocin use is rare.

In this active management protocol, monitoring is used to avoid fetal distress. In the original active management protocol, oxytocin as a medical treatment was not used in the multiparous patient for fear of uterine rupture.[10] It was inferred in this treatment plan that poor forces of labor were the problems with most abnormal labors, and cephalo-pelvic disproportion could be ruled out and avoided by trial of labor. Most multiparas will manage these problems spontaneously without the use of oxytocin. As suggested by Cardozo et al.[13] problems of position, such as rotation (occiput posterior, occiput transverse), deflexion, and descent, are secondary to inadequate uterine forces.

In this text, adherence to a protocol of "active labor management" is not urged. However, intervening earlier and more frequently with oxytocin augmentation is an individualized patient care theme. The use of oxytocin in all patients, including multiparous women, is acceptable. It is understood that with increasing parity and uterine size, prudent judgment associated with this treatment mode must be exercised according to the individual patient.

Most clinicians use modifications of this "active labor management" approach. Individualized patient management is offered. Use all the potential treatment measures, including time, ambulation, membrane rupture, and oxytocin. The Friedman system documents what is happening at any moment in time better than the arbitrary 1 cm/hr guideline for dilatation. Admitting patients later in latent-phase or active-phase labor, and anticipating slow or faster time periods for cervical dilatation and vertex descent, is part of the plan offered in this text.

Summary

1. Neurologic pathology following difficult labors, defined as protractions or arrests, has not decreased with the increased use of cesarean in dystocia.

2. The term *dystocia* is a vague descriptor for a difficult labor and should be discarded for more descriptive terms.

3. Terms such as *cephalo-pelvic disproportion, failure of forces, uterine inertia,* and *dysfunctional labor* should no longer be used as labor diagnoses without adequate description of the rationale for their use.

4. Labor should be described in terms of latent, active, and second stages, with normal or abnormal progress described as protractions or arrests of dilatation or descent.

References

1. Moloy HC. Clinical and Roentgenologic Evaluation of the Pelvis in Obstetrics. Philadelphia, WB Saunders, 1951 (foreword by HC Taylor, Jr).

2. Shiono PH, McNellis DM, Rhoads CC. Reasons for the rising cesarean delivery rates 1978–84. Obstet Gynecol 1987;69:696–700.

3. Shiono PH, Ficiden JG, McNeflis D, et al. Recent trends in cesarean birth and trial of labor rates in the U.S. JAMA 1987;257:494–497.

4. Bottoms SF, Hirsch VJ, Sokol RJ. Medical management of arrest disorders of labor a current overview. Am J Obstet Gynecol 1987;156:935–939.

5. Rosen MG, Debanne SM, Thompson K. Arrest disorders and infant brain damage. Obstet Gynecol 1989;74:300–324.

6. Cesarean Childbirth, Bethesda, MD, National Institutes of Health, Publication 82-2067, October 1981, pp 159–239.

7. Gross TL, Sokol RS, King KC. Obesity and pregnancy: Risks and outcomes. Obstet Gynecol 1980;56:446–450.

8. Thomas H. Pelvimetry. New York, Paul B. Hoeber, Inc, 1956, p 9.

9. Acker DB, Sachs BP, Friedman EA. Risk factors for shoulder dystocia. Obstet Gynecol 1985;66:762–768.

10. Cohen WR. The influence of the duration of the second stage of labor on perinatal outcome and perceptual morbidity. Obstet Gynecol 1977;49:266–269.

11. O'Driscoll K, Foley M, MacDonald D. Active management of labour as an alternative to cesearean section. Obstet Gynecol 1984;63:485–490.

12. Philpott RH. The recognition of cephalopelvic disproportion. Clin Obstet Gynecol 1982;9:609–624.

13. Cardozo LD, Gibbs DMF, Shedd JW, et al. Predictive value of cerviocometric labor patterns in primigravidae. Br J Obstet Gynaecol 1982;89:33–38.

Chapter 10

Cesarean Delivery

Overview

In recent years the incidence of delivery by cesarean section has risen to over 25% of all deliveries. The reasons for this increase are multiple. The advent of electronic monitoring has certainly increased the diagnosis of "fetal distress" and thus has been a large component of the rise.[1] Other factors include the almost routine delivery of all breeches by cesarean section, the medicolegal concerns of the physician in the patient with any perceived abnormality of the fetus, and the ever increasing diagnosis of "failure to progress." On a case-by-case basis, it is difficult to fault any of these rationales, however, when applied to obstetricians in general, there is increasing concern that this operation is occurring too frequently. On the other hand, what is the right proportion is still unknown and unproven.

Objectives

At the conclusion of this chapter the clinician should.

1. Know the most common indications for cesarean delivery
2. Recognize the appropriate methods of cesarean delivery
3. Understand the common complications and their management
4. Have the basic knowledge necessary to evaluate the diagnosis of and alternative measures for management of patients considered for cesarean section

Details

Indications

Cesarean delivery should be performed as an alternative to vaginal delivery only when there is a clear indication that the fetus or the mother is in jeopardy, or when there is an inability of the fetus to deliver through the vagina. In each of these instances, the record should clearly document the diagnosis and rationale behind the diagnosis. Although there will be subjective evaluation of the available information, objective data should be the focal point.

The most common indication for a primary cesarean section is cephalo-pelvic disproportion (CPD). This diagnosis occurs in up to 40% of all primary cesarean deliveries. As the name implies, it occurs when the fetal skull is too large to pass through the pelvic structures. This may be the result of a large head in the fetus or a narrowing of the pelvic architecture, especially the midplane, in the mother. To be truly diagnosed, the cervix should be completely dilated for a period of 2 hours in a patient with ruptured membranes and adequate labor. (Evaluation of the patient will often reveal excessive caput formation as well as an inability to move the vertex further into the pelvis by use of abdominal compression.) These classical findings are adhered to too infrequently on most obstetrical units, and thus the diagnosis is made on the basis of clinical judgment at an earlier stage.

EXAMPLE

Mrs. J., a 29-year-old primigravida, began labor at 2:00 am. She was admitted at 4:00 am at 3 cm, 100% effaced, and –2 station. After 8 hours of labor she had progressed to complete dilation, but the presenting vertex was at –1 station. One hour later she was still in active labor with the presenting part at +1 station. Her physician made the diagnosis of CPD and delivered a 7 lb 3oz infant by cesarean section.

Comment

(Although this patient had an uneventful course she received less than optimal care.) Without any other rationale requiring immediate delivery, her physician based his diagnosis on the fact that the patient had not made sufficient descent and thus, by exclusion, CPD must be present. There are many factors that cause a delay in descent with active labor. Each of these must be evaluated, and if progress is made, even slowly, then CPD is difficult to establish.

An emerging major diagnosis for primary cesarean delivery is "failure to progress." This is a diagnosis that was almost unheard of 20 to 40 years ago and now is a common justification for abdominal delivery. The definition is as elusive as the diagnosis. For most clinicians it means that the normal progression of labor has plateaued. It may be a precursor of CPD, it may reflect inefficient or insufficient uterine contractions, it may reflect fetal malposition, or it may occur for other reasons. Regardless, it is not a distinct entity and thus must be carefully evaluated before being accepted. When labor slows, the obstetrician must reexamine and reevaluate the patient. Correction of any adverse findings may solve the problem without requiring operative intervention.[3] Previous discussion in prior chapters has explained this problem more completely.

EXAMPLE

A 24-year-old primigravida was admitted in active labor at 5 cm and +1 station. Three hours later she was 6 cm dilated with contractions every 5 minutes, lasting 30 seconds. The diagnosis of "failure to progress" was made, and abdominal delivery was performed. Obviously this patient's progress was slow, but before any diagnosis was made adequate evaluation as well as improvement of contractions was necessary.

With the advent of electronic fetal monitoring, continuous evaluation of the fetal heart rate became a reality. As a result, the diagnosis of fetal heart-rate abnormalities became possible.[1] Based on this information, the next step was to interpret patterns of fetal distress and use this information to determine conditions requiring the performance of emergency or urgent cesarean delivery for fetal reasons. The diagnosis of fetal distress has improved over the years, and we now recognize patterns of "stress", non-reassuring patterns, baseline abnormalities, as well as placental abnormalities. Unfortunately, interpretation of the various patterns has not been a precise science, and two "experts" viewing the same pattern can have different interpretations. This has led to numerous lawsuits but has not been shown to have a major impact on lowering perinatal mortality.[1,3] Reliance on clinical judgment is still the best method to manage a patient in labor. The electronic fetal monitor is but one of the several clinical tools that can assist in this judgment.

There are few strictly maternal reasons for cesarean delivery. Most of the medical complications can be managed medically and allow the patient to tolerate labor. Malignancy, especially of the reproductive tract, is one such indication. Others include placental abnormalities such as a placenta previa, vasa previa, or an abruption. Rare instances of vaginal tumors or other obstructions have been reported, but for most clinicians these are never seen in a practice.

Methods

Abdominal delivery is usually performed by one of three methods: low transverse, classical, or extraperitoneal. The most common technique in the United States is low transverse. In this technique the bladder is removed from the lower uterine segment and the incision is made in a transverse fashion. Over 90% of incisions are made in this fashion because it has less blood loss, less adhesion formation, and allows for vaginal delivery in subsequent pregnancies. A variation in a small number of cases is a vertical incision. However, this often extends into the uterine muscle and thus has problems similar to a classical incision.

The classical incision is a vertical incision made in the midline of the corpus. It is infrequently performed but may be the incision of choice for a transverse lie, placenta previa, or in the presence of extensive adhesions. Some physicians also believe it will allow a more rapid entry into the uterus, but this is not universal. In subsequent pregnancies, the risk of uterine rupture, even before labor, is much higher with this incision.

Extraperitoneal incisions are extremely rare. They were previously used to reduce intraabdominal infections, but in modern-day obstetrics they are not indicated. Most obstetricians have never seen one, much less performed one.

Complications

As with any surgical procedure, cesarean section is not without complications. There are the complications related to the surgery itself, such as entry into the bowel or bladder, injury to the uterine vessels, dehiscence of the incision, ileus, and thromboembolism. There is also the ever-present potential of infection, both in the uterus and in the incision. Because this operation is so common, we often forget its hazards. It is important to realize that the morbidity and mortality of cesarean section is real and omnipresent. Therefore, these risks must be considered and evaluated prior to making the decision to operate.

Summary

Cesarean section is second only to episiotomy as the most common operation in obstetrics. Any clinician who does obstetrics will inevitably have a patient who needs abdominal delivery. However, before proceeding the following points must be considered:

1. Adequate evaluation prior to making a diagnosis is essential.
2. The most common indication is cephalo-pelvic disproportion.
3. The preferred method is a low transverse cervical approach.
4. There are risks and complications, including injury and infection, that must be considered.

References

1. American College of Obstetricians and Gynecologists. Fetal Heart Rate Patterns: Monitoring, Interpretation and Management. Technical Bulletin #207. Washington, DC, ACOG, July, 1995.
2. Colditz PB, Henderson-Smart DJ. Electronic fetal heart rate monitoring during labor. Does it prevent perinatal asphyxia and cerebral palsy? Med J Austral 1990;153: 88–90.
3. Lagrew DC, Morgan MA. Decreasing the cesarean section rate in a private hospital: Success without mandated clinical change. Am J Obstet Gynecol 1996;174:184–91.

Chapter 11

Forceps
Practical Considerations

Overview

Almost from the moment forceps were invented, their use — or misuse — was debated. Today, forceps should remain an acceptable choice for the trained obstetrician. Midforceps may also be used, but the term *midforceps* cannot be separated into terms such as difficult or easy midforceps, or even low midforceps. If low forceps are used, inevitably midforceps will be used on the occasion in which a strict criteria for the definition of low forceps is not applied. The physician tends to describe forceps as lower in classification because of the negative comments that often follow the term *mid* associated with forceps. The term *midforceps* is also very broad. For example, a midforceps performed from station +1 is far more difficult when compared with a midforceps performed at station +3 or +4 in a five-station pelvis.

In this chapter, the evolution of forceps is reviewed, and the origins of the midforceps debate is described. Findings relating infant outcome to midforceps use are presented. Finally, definitions for forceps classification are presented based on the station when the forceps were applied and the position of the vertex. The key principle in this chapter is the use of clinical judgment. There are choices in clinical care, and there is no need to return to difficult and traumatic deliveries.

Objectives

At the conclusion of this chapter the physician should be able to

1. Present definitions for forceps classification
2. Replace terms such as *midforceps* or *low forceps* with the new classification based on the pelvic station at which forceps are applied
3. Understand the guidelines for forceps use

4. Discuss basic type of forceps and understand some technical considerations in forcep use

A Brief History of Forceps

Claude Heaton, waxing poetic in the preface to Dennen's classic monograph *Forceps Deliveries,* wrote, "the obstetrical forceps has been described as a noble and beneficent instrument rescuing more lives and cutting short more pains than all other instruments in the professional armamentarium." Heaton described the invention of forceps by Peter Chamberlen, Sr, A French Huguenot refugee who went to England in 1569. At first in secret, the use of forceps became well-known after Edmund Chapman published information on forceps use in 1733.[1] Obviously, not all clinicians were then or remain now as sanguine as Dr. Heaton about the use of these instruments for facilitating birth. Speert,[2] writing more conservatively of obstetrical interventions, presented a negative view: "Nature is the best judge in childbearing in a normal process; nature should be allowed to take its course." To paraphrase Speert, don't rush to use forceps or to intervene. Today this perspective is encouraged.

An even more negative approach to forceps use was reported in a review by Richardson et al. published in 1985.[3] Richardson quoted William Hunter's writing on forceps use in the mid-1700s. "It was a thousand pities (forceps) were invented, where they save one, they murder twenty." In the early 19th century, as a result of changing physician attitudes derived from the early misuse of forceps, they had all but been eliminated.[3] The classic triple tragedy known to all obstetricians exemplified a period of time when forceps use was not advocated. In that episode, fetal death occurred following a protracted labor, followed by Princess Charlotte's death. This was a labor in which forceps use may have saved either of the potential rulers of England. The alternative, the cesarean, would have been mortal for the future queen.[3]

As anesthesia, surgical technology, and understanding of infection advanced, the use of forceps returned. Dr. Joseph Clark, Master of the Rotunda between 1786 and 1793, reported average forceps use in one of 743 births.[3] In 1875, more than 100 years later, Dr. George Johnson, then Master of the Rotunda, reported a remarkably increased forceps rate of one in ten births.[3] Obviously attitudes towards this instrument had changed.

To a large degree, the use of forceps became universal in the 1900s when Delee, in 1921, advocated the prophylactic use of forceps to shorten the second stage of labor. This reflected the 2-hour rule discussed in earlier chapters. By 1951, Dieckman reported that 68% of all births at the Chicago Lying-In Hospital were facilitated with forceps.[3]

Throughout the history of forceps, almost seasonal advocacy or restriction of their use has continued. Duncan Reid[4] encouraged the use of oxytocin, thus leading to a decreased need for forceps use. In 1953, E. Steward Taylor[5] proposed elimination of midforceps because of their marked destructive effects on the mother and fetus. In the 1960s, under his stewardship, midforceps were all but eliminated at the University of Colorado in Denver.

Friedman et al.[6] suggested that protractions, arrests, and midforceps labors were associated with lower IQs in children at 7 years of age. In contrast to midforceps, low forceps did not show similar outcomes in the study. Friedman and Rosen debated this finding publicly. It should be noted that comparable births by cesarean following abnormal labors (the appropriate comparison population) were not studied in the Friedman report.

Today the question remains when abnormal labor is present, a finding that can only be diagnosed once it is present, how should the patient be delivered? The fetus must be born. Forceps trauma to the mother and fetus have been described in many studies. Comparable data on birth route by cesarean in the presence of abnormalities of labor randomly substituted for birth route by forceps are not available.

A second question still facing the clinician is whether the change in birth route, once the labor diagnosis has been made, will alter infant morbidity. To end this review, but not the debate, a report by Kadar and Romero[7] notes that 75% of instrumentally delivered primigravidas delivered heavier babies spontaneously in the next gestation. The authors also note that in the remainder of the population studied, operative delivery was six times greater than in the normal population. This suggests that the original midforceps group will be at risk for later labor difficulties, even though three out of four mothers may deliver fetuses spontaneously in the next birth. As noted in vaginal birth after cesarean studies, a second pregnancy usually correlates with a first pregnancy labor experience, and the normal outcomes exceed the problem outcomes.

Definitions and Terminology

Medical and legal implications associated with the term *midforceps* have led to changes in behavior and have often resulted in incorrect classification of the charted data by the physician. The terms *low forceps* and *midforceps* are extremely broad. The current terminology is presented to advocate the use of a more simple forceps classification, one based on pelvic station and vertex position as defined by the American College of Obstetricians and Gynecologists and illustrated in Table 11.1.[8,9]

Classification of Forceps by Pelvic Station and Vertex Position

Stations +3 and +4 are generally stations from which vaginal birth is expected. Vertex position, molding of the vertex, as well as maternal, fetal, and pelvic size

Table 11.1   Proposed Forceps Classification

Station	Vertex Position
0	OA, LOA, ROA, LOT, ROT, LOP, ROP, OP
+1	OA, LOA, ROA, LOT, ROT, LOP, ROP, OP
+2	OA, LOA, ROA, LOT, ROT, LOP, ROP, OP
+3	OA, LOA, ROA, LOT, ROT, LOP, ROP, OP
+4	OA, LOA, ROA, LOT, ROT, LOP, ROP, OP
+5	OA, LOA, ROA, LOT, ROT, LOP, ROP, OP

Abbreviations: O, occiput; A, anterior; L, left; R, right; T, transverse; P, posterior.

influence the physician's expectations. At these lower positions cesarean delivery may not be easily accomplished, as the lower uterine segment will be quite thin and fragile, and the low position of the vertex within the pelvis will necessitate force to return it to the abdomen. Many clinicians have spent a great deal of time resuturing the lower uterine segment, which literally falls apart after a long labor, following a difficult abdominal extraction of the fetus from a low pelvic station, performed in order to avoid use of forceps.

The new forceps descriptive terminology based on vertex station, and position, has several advantages. All reviewers will know what the operation means when the forceps are described as station S+2, vertex LOA. This statement describes not only pelvic position but also implies a degree of difficulty if forceps are used. Compare this statement to S+4, vertex LOA, and the conclusions are obvious. The clinician expects less difficulty or need for traction to be applied at a lower pelvic station. Furthermore, investigators reviewing charts and attempting to determine at what pelvic station forceps application may increase morbidity for mother of fetus, could compare pelvic stations and vertex positions. In most studies this information is not easily obtained. In many chart notes, forceps are often categorized as low or mid, yet pelvic station may not be mentioned.

Guidelines for Forceps Use

Station

If after vaginal examination, it is the clinician's judgment that the forceps birth will be difficult, even when it is known that the procedure can be accomplished, do not proceed. For obvious reasons, difficult forceps should be avoided unless, in the physician's judgment, cesarean birth or further time cannot be allowed. Forceps at station 0 and +1 are considered difficult and are generally replaced by allowing for more time in labor, if acceptable, or by cesarean if more time for labor is not acceptable. Station +2 is generally a transition point in the judgment for forceps use. Data relating to morbidity at different midpelvic stations are not available. Some obstetricians will deliver at this station; others feel that lack of experience does not allow a choice. Vertex position obviously should influence the decision. Forceps rotations from vertex positions other than the anterior position infer more difficulty.

Forceps use at stations +4 or +5 should be obvious. At those stations it is difficult to conceive of not delivering a vertex vaginally from any vertex position, including transverse and posterior. Station +4 should not be elective forceps use but warranted because of patient progress or fetal needs. Station +5 forceps use may be for various reasons, but it is primarily for maternal assistance.

Flexion

Flexion of the vertex facilitates passage of a smaller diameter of the vertex and foreshadows an easier birth. Without good flexion expect more difficulty. To flex the vertex with forceps is a procedure that must be taught in the delivery room. The position of the anterior and posterior fontanels, and whether the forceps blades at their heel or shanks are about two fingerbreadths below the posterior fontanel, need to be noted during forceps application. If the shanks of the forceps are not in this position, the clinician may flex the vertex by opening, reapplying, and depressing the forceps blades so that vertex will be flexed and come through the pelvis with a smaller diameter, therefore requiring less traction.

Asynclitism

Asynclitism, or lateral vertex flexion, is associated with a more difficult forceps application and more difficult delivery. Lateral flexion is corrected after the forceps application has begun. In contrast to actively flexing the head and changing the forceps position in a deflexed head, asynclitism is corrected as the forceps blades are applied while attempting to lock the blades. At this point, the clinician will find that one blade is higher on the vertex than its counterpart. Locking of the blades cannot take place until the forceps blades are manipulated to have equal length while correcting the lateral flexion of the vertex. If fenestrated forceps are being used, more of the fenestration (window) will be apparent on the side that must be deflexed. As the forceps blade is elevated and locked, the asynclitism is usually corrected. Asynclitism suggests more difficulty in forceps application and traction.

The Sacrum

If during the vaginal examination the hollow of the sacrum is easily felt behind the vertex, the vertex is either quite small or at much higher station than the operator anticipated. Discovering that there is room behind the vertex (in front of the sacrum) also implies that with further descent there should be more-room in the pelvis for the vertex.

Vertex Position

The position of the vertex must be known. Without knowledge of at least the sagittal suture position, safe forceps application cannot be performed. The presence of the fontanels most easily indicates fetal position. When in doubt, search for an ear higher along the side of the vertex. The resistance of the back of the ear may help define the direction of the occiput. If the maternal abdomen has been examined earlier in labor, useful information will have been obtained. The back may have been palpated and also visualized as the straight side. The back and occiput should be on the same side. The information obtained from these earlier examinations may confirm an uncertain vaginal examination.

Vertex Molding

The long molded head found following a labor with a protracted active phase or a prolonged second stage should suggest that the vertex is at a higher pelvic station than it feels by palpation. A greater degree of difficult with forceps use may be expected. Patients need to be evaluated in the context of the total labor picture, not just isolated pieces of information, such as pelvic station or cervical dilatation.

Cervical Dilatation

The cervix must be fully dilated prior to applying forceps. In some cases the cervix will not disappear before vertex rotation takes place. The presence of a cervical rim or any palpable cervix along the side of the vertex suggests a more difficult procedure. Forceps use in these situations should be uncommon.

Fetal Size

The size of the fetus should be estimated by manual examination or by ultrasonography. Fetal size in general terms (large, average, or small) should have been estimated earlier in labor, when the chart note was first written and the patient's labor was evaluated.

Pelvic Size

As stated earlier in this text, clinical estimation of pelvic size has been scorned by many clinicians and urged by others. At the first prenatal encounter with the patient, a pelvic estimate in general terms should be made. While the limitations of these measurements are understood, some general estimate is useful. In the delivery room, prior to forceps application, again attempt to review the patients' size and her clinical pelvimetry in association with the position of the vertex. These parameters are more meaningful if they are performed long before the patient's labor becomes complicated.

Clinical Indications for Forceps Use

In the previous section on guidelines for forceps use, some general assumptions were presented regarding information that should be known prior to the use of forceps. In this section on clinical indications for forceps, appropriate situations are presented when clinical choices and judgment, based on findings, come into play.

Fetal Distress

Fetal distress is an acceptable indication for forceps intervention. If, in the operator's judgment, fetal distress is present and some intervention should take place, the choice of forceps is acceptable. The clinical principles mentioned earlier apply. The sum of an equation, which balances fetal distress and potential trauma, needs to include an estimation of how serious the fetal distress may be, how rapidly the baby should be extracted (either by cesarean or forceps), and how difficult the forceps procedure is expected to be.

EXAMPLE OF POSSIBLE UMBILICAL CORD COMPRESSION

Following a normal labor, a primigravid patient was 35 minutes into the second stage, fully dilated, with membranes ruptured, and at S+3 and vertex OA. Severe variable decelerations followed each contraction. The fetus was average in size. Clinical pelvimetry was felt to be normal. A fetal scalp blood sample revealed a mild respiratory acidosis with pH 7.21. Despite these findings, heart-rate beat-to-beat variability appeared to be diminishing and the operator was concerned.

Comments

Although the situation was not yet critical, it was worrisome. Choices included waiting and repeating the scalp blood test, performing a cesarean, the use of midforceps, or vacuum extraction. The operator, believing the delivery to be relatively easy, chose to use Simpson forceps along with local anesthesia over a midline episiotomy. This clinical judgment is acceptable. The use of the vacuum or repetition of the scalp blood test would have been acceptable alternatives. There was no reason for a cesarean.

In some hospitals cesareans may be accomplished within 5 to 15 minutes from the time the crisis is detected. This level of support allows the clinician greater flexibility in treatment of choice. A forceps at station 0 may easily be replaced by a cesarean in the operator's judgment. In contrast, if 30 minutes or longer is required to effect delivery, the clinician's judgment of fetal risk may warrant vaginal forceps birth at most pelvic stations below +1.

In describing acute situations such as fetal distress associated with abruption of the placenta or umbilical cord prolapse in the second stage of labor, once again evaluation of the reasons for the problem precedes clinical judgment and management. Although in this case forceps use is being discussed, in another instance the etiology of acute fetal distress may alter the clinician's consideration. A prolapsed umbilical cord may be treated first by vertex displacement, which may allow the operator more time to make a decision regarding a birth route choice. A placental separation is a very different problem.

Labor Abnormalities

In the presence of labor abnormalities, when time in seconds or minutes is not as critical, clinical judgment may be somewhat different. In labor abnormality situations, awaiting descent to lower stations and allowing more time in labor often will answer the problem and avoid the more difficult forceps. The difficult labor, followed by a forceps applied at stations +2 or +3, may foreshadow much more fetal risk than allowing an additional period of time to await further vertex descent. An arrest of descent at station +2 or +3 implies no similar urgency; this is in contrast to fetal distress, a situation in which length of time until delivery may be critical.

Arrest of Descent

The second stage of labor eventually must end, but, 1- or 2-hour time limits are arbitrary endpoints. Rather, the question should be whether progress is continuing or has descent arrested. If progress is continuing and time is not a problem (fetal distress is not present), the answer is easily reached: Wait longer! If the patient needs more pain relief, use it.

Elective Forceps

Elective forceps is not an acceptable term. The use of forceps at any station is associated with some maternal and fetal risk. The term *elective* implies no presenting urgency for birth from maternal or fetal indications. If a mother is exhausted and the vertex is at station +4 or station +5, that is not an elective forceps use. Exhaustion needs treatment, and forceps use or regional anesthesia are appropriate treatment choices.

In contrast, if epidural anesthesia has been given and rotation and descent appear to have ceased, then oxytocin, or allowing the epidural block to wear off, are more acceptable choices prior to forceps application.

Teaching Forceps

Teaching forceps is also an unacceptable term; appropriate judgment should be taught. Forceps should not be applied electively in order to teach a resident. In those instances poor judgment is being taught. The less frequent use of forceps in obstetrics suggest that experience in the use of forceps should be more focused in the later years of resident education. Forceps use above station +4 should only be performed by residents in their senior years.

The number of forceps experiences that are needed by the resident in order to become comfortable and skilled in their use is a concern. The appropriate analogy is that the gynecology resident may perform 10, 15, or 25 vaginal hysterectomies before being considered adequately educated. Forceps experience depends on particular clinical conditions. Because forceps are less commonly used, their use must be taught well when it occurs. They should not be performed without the presence of an experienced clinician. All too often resident education is passed on from one resident to the next. Forceps use in many environments is too infrequent an occurrence to accept this learning method. Perhaps the learning of forceps should be treated with the same concern as the learning of difficult surgery. Certainly, the implications in forceps use warrants this consideration.

Low-BirthWeight Fetus

The small fetus, categorized as the low-birthweight (<2500 g) or very low-birthweight (<1500 g) fetus, has been involved in the forceps debate for many years. Initially the debate involved the use of forceps in babies weighing 4 or 5 lb. It was never established whether, at those low birthweights, placing the fetal vertex in a "cage" to protect it from vaginal pressure or from too rapid expansion of the skull at birth produced improved results. Today, the data indicating forceps use for the very low-birthweight fetus of less than 1500 g are even more limited. Forceps should be applied only if delivery needs to be effected because of clinical circumstances. Forceps are not a routine part of the care for the low-birthweight fetus.

Even more controversial in this very low-birthweight group is the suggestion by some clinicians that cesarean birth should be performed to improve fetal outcome and to prevent trauma or intracerebral fetal hemorrhage. At this time, there are no acceptable data documenting improved fetal outcome resulting from the cesarean birth route in the very low-birthweight group. Birth of this more fragile fetus requires attention, the presence of an experienced clinician, and a controlled delivery. This is the best clinical advice that can be offered until controlled studies are performed that test the hypothesis that change in birth route will improve outcome for the very low-birthweight fetus.

The attempt to apply forceps to a low-birthweight fetus is more easily decided upon than performed. When trying to apply forceps during a rapidly progressing labor, fetal position is often confusing. In the low-birthweight fetus, because of the large fontanels and the soft skull, uncertainty of fetal position may lead to an attempt to apply forceps either too soon or too late. If applied too soon, there is a temptation to deliver the fetus from a higher station, and that is unacceptable. If applied too late, the head is born before the clinician is prepared. The important principle in birth technique for the low-birthweight fetus is to control the rapidity of the birth of the head. This is effected by the presence of adequate perineal room provided by an episiotomy. The vertex should be born gradually, not abruptly. The clinician's hands should remain on the fetal vertex throughout the birth, and they should guide and control the descent and extension of the crowning vertex. It is not only vaginal muscle pressure on the fetal vertex that is a concern, but also too rapid expansion of the bones of the skull. If the head is born too rapidly, intracranial hemorrhage, such as dural sinus lacerations, may occur. However, intracerebral bleeding in the low-birthweight fetus appears to be more related to fetal maturity than to birth route choice.

Technical Considerations in Forceps Use

Techniques for procedures such as forceps delivery or breech birth are best taught in the delivery room. In the discussions on forceps, a philosophy and guideline for judgment has been presented. However, some statements may be made about the technical use of the forceps.

Types of Forceps

Since the use of forceps in most hospitals has been replaced with other methodologies, such as a tincture of time, the cesarean, or the vacuum extractor, technical skills are best acquired with simplified and standardized approaches to forceps use, which may be repeated more frequently. If Barton's or Kielland's forceps are rarely used, it is unlikely that adequate skill and confidence with these instruments will be retained. It is suggested that forceps use be limited to a few frequently used types.

A Simpson-type forceps with separated and parallel shanks should be appropriate for almost all births of the term-size fetus during labor. For the smaller fetus, or the nonmolded fetal vertex, forceps with overlapping shanks will serve the rounder or smaller vertex. Rotations may be performed with these same forceps. If, in the clinician's judgment, the vertex position is too difficult to consider use of a Simpson-type forceps, it may perhaps be best not to use any forceps.

EXAMPLE OF BARTON FORCEPS OR NO FORCEPS

At term a normal-sized fetus presented with the cervix fully dilated, vertex LOT, station +2, and with a posterior parietal asynclitism. The Barton's forceps (with the anterior hinged blade) would have been an ideal instrument for delivery in this presentation.

Comment

Today, few clinicians can apply, rotate, and use traction with Barton's forceps. Because Barton's forceps are used infrequently, it may be best not to teach their use. Perhaps a vacuum extraction would be appropriate. Perhaps more time is needed. Appropriate forceps choice may be accomplished with a classical Simpson-type forceps, or if immediate delivery is warranted, a cesarean may be less traumatic than forceps. This is a judgment of the clinician's and, in part, depends on previous thinking.

Forceps Traction

Axis traction instruments are not recommended. If downward pressure on the forceps shanks and outward traction from the handle (known as the Pajot-Saxtorph maneuver) (Fig. 11.1) does not allow descent of the vertex under the symphysis, perhaps too much force may be needed and the procedure should be reconsidered. The use of an axis traction instrument allows a great deal of force to be used without the operator sensing it during the traction.

Pelvic Curve and the Director of Forceps Traction

To use traction, an understanding of the sacral pelvic curve with flexing of the occiput under the symphysis pubis is needed prior to extension of the vertex over the perineum. It is a common error for the operator to sit at the foot of the delivery table and, after the forceps application, apply horizontal traction towards the operator (Fig. 11.2A,B). This is obviously incorrect. The downward pressure on the forceps shanks (Fig. 11.2C) modulated with the horizontal traction toward the operator allows vertex descent toward the floor, under the pubic symphysis, and the force vector or correct direction of the applied forces is achieved.

The ability to balance these two operator-applied forces allows a controlled vertex birth. At higher stations the operator must first use greater downward pressure on the forceps shanks. If during traction, particularly during forceps at stations +2 or +3, appropriate direction of the vertex under the symphysis pubis is not accomplished, greater force is required and greater pressure of the pubic symphysis on the skull occurs. Note again that these techniques are best taught in the delivery room when the delivery forces can be felt by the operator. Even the sitting position of the clinician on a stool at the foot of the delivery table is more easily understood when described in the delivery room. At that time the operator will understand why sitting on a low stool allows more efficient forceps traction at stations of the pelvis above +4 and +5.

Trial and Failed Forceps

These two terms represent a final attitude in a philosophy about forceps. If forceps are applied and it is discovered unexpectedly that they cannot be correctly applied, or after application in the delivery of the vertex in the operator's judgment acceptable traction is exceeded, it is wise to stop. That is a failed forceps. To the less experienced obstetrician, how hard to pull with forceps and what is an acceptable application must be learned under the supervision of an experienced clinician. After several forceps applications, norms for acceptable traction are learned.

A procedure approached such as "trial forceps" suggests uncertainty and anticipation of difficulty before starting. Reevaluate the situation. It does not take a great deal of humility to decide that more time in labor, oxytocin use, anesthesia, or a cesarean may be appropriate. A trial of forceps should be a very uncommon approach to patient care.

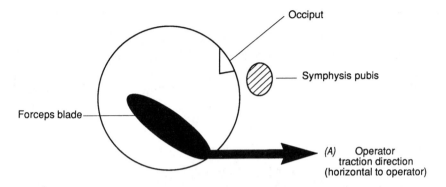

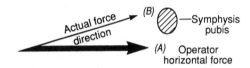

If traction is pulled towards the operator (A), the effective force (B) drives the occiput into the symphysis pubis. This is unacceptable.

A way must be found to direct the vertex <u>under</u> the pubic symphysis. This is found by adding a second force (C) perpendicular to the floor that now changes the direction of the vertex (B).

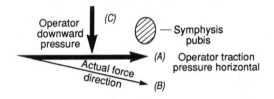

FIGURE 11.1

Data from the Cleveland Midforceps Program

To attempt to rationalize the problem — to use or not to use the midforceps — the data from Cleveland Metropolitan General Hospital during the late 1970s and early 1980s was reviewed.[10] At that hospital midforceps application was acceptable, but it was urged that midforceps use be performed with an experienced physician present, with caution, and in general at lower pelvic stations. The term *elective midforceps* was not used. There was no "teaching" midforceps use. Midforceps were performed primarily for arrests or protractions in the second stage of labor at midpelvic stations or for fetal distress. The judgment to use midforceps, as taught by the faculty, was to neither "look for trouble" nor to try to demonstrate unusual technical skill. Rather, prior to forceps use, it was up to the physician to judge if, in a patient at a particular pelvic station, forceps use was a safe alternative birth for mother and fetus.

Retrospective studies compared infant outcome between cesarean birth and forceps delivery. The outcome variable sought was major infant brain damage. Data were collected from matched infant chart notes with similar labor diagnoses. The hypothesis was that in the restricted approach to midforceps, their use was not associated with increased risk for mother or infant. This hypothesis could not be disproved. The meaning of "restricted" becomes more apparent when it is noted that the incidence of midforceps use was less than 1% of all births. Forceps applications at stations 0 and +1 were not encouraged, and pelvic station +2 was borderline for decision-making when using the five pelvic stations.

The findings documented that there was a significantly higher rate of active-phase and second-stage labor abnormalities in the midforceps-use group than in the general population. This was understandable since therapeutic interventions, such as patience, sedation, ambulation, position change, membrane rupture, and oxytocin use, were encouraged before considering the "ending" of labor by forceps or cesarean.

Latent-phase labor abnormalities were not significantly increased in the midforceps-use group when compared with all other patients, demonstrating once again that terminating a labor in latent phase is generally not an adequate trial for vaginal birth, and that a prolonged latent phase does not predict a difficult active phase or abnormal second stage of labor. No increase in midforceps use in the over 4000-g fetuses was found. Midforceps use in excessive size infants was not encouraged.

Short-term neonatal morbidity, including depressed Apgar scores, seventh nerve palsy, and neonatal seizures, were found to be the same for both midforceps and cesarean birth infants born with the same labor abnormalities. The midforceps group did exhibit a higher incidence of cephalohematoma.

Continuing this study of infants born between 1976 and 1982, through the first 2 years of life, matching the use of forceps for labor abnormality or for fetal distress, no significant difference in infant abnormal neurologic development were found.[4] While these two studies obviously did not end the debate, they at least allowed for the generalizations made about midforceps use.

The Vacuum Extractor

The nonrigid soft vacuum extraction instrument is currently in use in most areas of the country. Vacuum extraction of a fetus must be considered another mechanical traction instrument. It is useful, but it is not harmless. In general, indications for its use are similar to those of forceps. It is interesting to note that some reports document the use of the vacuum at higher stations and, on occasion, through an incompletely dilated cervix.[10,11]

Broekhuizen et al.[12] noted vacuum extractions were being performed at higher stations — 59.8% at station +1 or higher — compared with only 9% of forceps being used at similar stations. There appeared to be less maternal trauma, although fetal skull fracture rates were similar when compared with forceps use at similar stations. The infants had a higher incidence of shoulder dystocia in the vacuum group. The major point to be made about the vacuum extractor is that while it is an acceptable technique to use, if indications for its use are expanded into areas already relinquished by forceps use, new data on morbidity will have to be collected. A conservative and less interventionist approach is suggested for the vacuum extractor, as with forceps.

Summary

1. Forceps and the vacuum extractor are acceptable parts of obstetrical treatment.

2. Classification of forceps by station and position of the vertex should replace terminology for midforceps, low midforceps, low forceps, and outlet forceps.

3. Classification of forceps by five stations of the pelvis allows for comparison among forceps of comparable difficulty.

4. Forceps performed at stations and +1 should be rare. The usually accepted transition point for forceps use appears to be pelvic station +2. It should be within the skills of the clinician to make a judgment choice for vaginal birth at stations +3, +4, and +5.

5. Forceps intervention should only be a final method for birth following appropriate labor trial or in the presence of fetal distress.

6. Forceps or cesarean birth are categories for terminating labor to be considered after other treatment modalities, such as time, ambulation, analgesia, oxytocin, and membrane rupture, have all been considered.

7. Midforceps use was more common when cesareans were not an available birth route choice.

8. During the early years of their use, midforceps led to many traumatic injuries to mother and fetus.

9. Changes in technology led to the replacement of difficult midforceps with the cesarean.

10. Neither prophylactic forceps use during the second stage of labor nor the 2-hour rule arose from data that warranted their application as dogma.

11. The introduction of the vacuum extractor should not be a license to perform more difficult mechanical deliveries.

References

1. Dennen EA: Forceps Deliveries. Philadelphia, FA Davis, 1955.

2. Speert H: Obstetrics and Gynecology in America: A History. Baltimore, Waverly Press, 1980, p 38.

3. Richardson DA, Evans M, Cibils L: Midforceps delivery: a critical review. Am J Obstet Gynecol 1983;145:621–632.

4. Reid DE: Treatment of prolonged labor with posterior pituitary extract. Am J Obstet Gynecol 1946;52:719–734.

5. Taylor ES: Can midforceps operations be eliminated. Obstet Gynecol 1953;2: 302–307.

6. Friedman EA, Sachtleben MR, Dahrouge D, Neff R: Long-term effects of labor and delivery on offspring: a matched pair analysis. Am J Obstet Gynecol 1984; 150:941–945.

7. Kadar N, Romero R: Prognosis for future childbearing after midcavity instrumental deliveries in primigravidas. Obstet Gynecol 1983;62:166–170.

8. Committee in Obstetrics. Maternal and Fetal Medicine. Obstetric Forceps Committee Opinion Paper No. 59, American College of Obstetricians and Gynecologists, Washington DC: February, 1988.

9. American College of Obstetricians and Gynecologists. Operative Vaginal delivery. ACOG Technical Bulletin 196. Washington DC, ACOG, 1994.

10 Dierker LJ, Rosen MG, Debanne S, Thompson K. The midforcep: Maternal and neonatal outcomes. Am J Obstet Gynecol 1985;152:176–183.

11. Dierker LJ, Rosen MG, Thompson K, Linn P. Midforceps—long-term outcome of infants. Am J Obstet Gynecol 1986;154:764–768.

12. Broekhuizen F, Washington J, Johnson F, Hamilton P. Vacuum extraction versus forceps delivery: Indications and complications, 1979–1984. Obstet Gynecol 1987; 69:338–342.

Chapter 12

Breech Presentation
The Controversy

An Overview

Perhaps even more controversial than forceps use is the problem of choice of route for delivery for the breech presentation. It is clouded by emotions, including physician and patient anxieties, and confusion of outcome benefit as recorded in the literature. By 1981 in the United States more than 60% of all fetuses in breech position were delivered by cesarean.[1] This increasing trend toward cesarean birth for the breech presentation has continued well beyond the time of this 1981 National Institutes of Health report.[1] It is apparent at most institutions that if the mother can be taken to the operating room before vaginal birth occurs, the cesarean will be the birth route. There is also a movement by some hospital risk-management personnel to urge the use of the cesarean birth route to avoid any potential litiginous consequences that may surround a breech fetus born vaginally. As in the cases of midforceps for fetal distress in a breech birth if morbidity develops during infancy or later in life, a search for etiology often returns to the birth process, even when data may suggest the birth process was not the problem.

The goal in this chapter is to demonstrate that, with respect to the breech presentation in labor, there is room for choice. It is important to understand why controversy exists and why choice of birth route is acceptable. To this end, the confounding variables in breech presentations that may make breech presentation an at-risk situation are explored first. A breech presentation may also be associated with non-birth-route incurred risks for neurological morbidity.

Objectives

At the conclusion of this section, the clinician should

1. Be aware of the literature describing birth route decisions for the breech presentation

2. Know the variables that will confuse outcome in all breech presentations
3. Be able to individualize patient care in reaching a birth-route choice in the frank breech position

Confounding Variables in the Breech Presentation That Lead to Increased Infant Morbidity and Morality

Certain risks cannot be altered by changing the birth route. The question that should be considered by the clinician prior to making a birth route decision is, Why is this fetus in breech presentation? At times the breech presentation may represent an already present fetal neurologic problem that has altered fetal movement patterns or body shape.

Congenital Anomalies and Abnormalities

Major anomalies of the fetus are severalfold higher in breech presentations.[2] Examples are Potters syndrome, with its abnormal fetal shape and absent kidneys, or congenital hydrocephalus, with its enlarged fetal head. These examples are two among many conditions that have a higher than anticipated risk for breech presentation. Prior to reaching a clinical decision for birth route, ultrasonography is necessary for fetal evaluation.[3] For example, in a fetus without kidneys it would not be prudent to deliver that breech position fetus by cesarean if vaginal birth were possible without incurring harm to the mother.

In contrast to gross congenital anomalies, it is also documented that the normal-appearing fetus in breech presentation has a higher than expected incidence of genetically acquired mental and biochemical abnormalities.[4] These gene abnormalities cannot be seen with ultrasonography but add to the already higher morbidity for the fetus in breech presentation.

Fetal Activity and Neurologic Function

More subtle and even more difficult to document is the thesis that fetal movement may be different in the breech presentation. In this speculation it is assumed that an already present neurologic abnormality makes the breech presentation fetus move differently from the vertex-presenting fetus. This infers that some developmental or traumatic event has taken place in the central nervous system prior to labor onset and delivery. For the obstetrician this documentation is usually made after delivery, if at all.

Prematurity

As the fetus approaches term, the incidence of breech presentation decreases. In the low-birthweight population, a higher incidence of the breech presentation is present, and infant outcome is intertwined with the risks of gestational immaturity. This is described more extensively in the following sections.

Other Confounding Variables

In association with low birthweight, we also find *premature rupture of the membranes* and *in utero infection* at higher incidence in the breech presentation. These obstetrical problems lead to higher morbidity and mortality irrespective of fetal position or birth route choice. Adding to the confusion, in many breech studies, which usually are reviews of a hospital's activities, the *stillbirth fetus* in breech presentation is always delivered vaginally. The live fetus in breech presentations is delivered by cesarean, again biasing some of the study numbers.

As opinions change and vaginal breech delivery returns as an option, newer management methods enter the confusing picture. The use of tocolytics and ultrasound have added to our ability to attempt to alter the breech position. Most significant has become the reemergence of the external cephalic version. Success rates as high as 65% have been reported.[5] This success has reduced the cesarean delivery rate significantly. Thus there is now one very significant confounding variable to be considered, and the obstetrician is left without a clear mandate but a clinical decision.

Risk Variables Intrinsic to the Breech Presentation During Labor

Fetal size, as in the large fetus is a concern in all gestations, but is even more worrisome in the breech presentation. Concern for difficulty in extracting the fetal shoulders or fetal head lead most clinicians to consider cesarean birth.

Similarly, in the small fetus a disproportionately large head compared with abdomen and shoulder size increases the concern for fetal-head entrapment. A small presenting part that does not fill the pelvis will increase the risk for prolapse of the umbilical cord. In comparison with the earlier confounding variables; these risks are associated primarily with vaginal birth, in the breech presentation some risks, such as prolapsed a umbilical cord, may occur quite early in labor onset, occurring with spontaneous membrane rupture even before the patient reaches the hospital.

Debate in the Literature

Hall et al.[6] reviewed the breech presentation and perinatal mortality over a 10-year period beginning in 1950. The authors presented data during a time when physicians' attitudes were evolving toward more frequent use of cesareans for many obstetrical problems. These authors noted the high incidence of low-birthweight fetuses in the breech category. Twenty-four to 30% of all breech presentations weighed between 1000 and 2500 g. The authors also confirmed that in the second 5 years of their report there was a 50% increase in breech cesarean birthrate, reaching a high of 15.1% of births by cesarean for the breech fetus. The high perinatal loss in the study associated with breech presentation was in part accounted for by low birthweight. In their conclusions, the authors stated that an increased risk for breech birth exists with vaginal birth, and urged the presence of an experienced physician when breech labor occurs.

In commenting on the paper by Hall et al.[6] which was presented at a meeting of the American Association of Obstetricians and Gynecologists in 1964, Robert A. Cosgrove noted his concern about the increasing use of cesareans for breech presentation, which resulted in cesarean sections 20% of the time at the Margaret Hague Maternity Hospital, where he was the director. These two commentaries documented the changing attitudes toward breech birth and the mixed judgment philosophies in this difficult obstetrical clinical decision.

Berendes et al.,[7] using sophisticated statistical approaches to the problem, attempted to determine the priority of importance of risk factors for both mortality and morbidity from the large number of breech births in the Collaborative Study of Cerebral Palsy. They found, among other risks, the strong influence of both congenital anomalies and birthweight on breech outcome.

By the mid-1970s most fetuses in breech presentation[8] were being delivered by cesarean. In a report by DeCrespigny and Pepperell, justification for the increased use of cesareans for the mature breech fetus (>2500 g) was questioned. The authors noted no increase in survival in the breech population when delivered by cesarean. Duenholter et al.,[9] in a controlled study during the same time period, suggested that the abdominal route was safer for the low-birthweight fetus (between 1000 and 2500 g). Discussing term infants, Mann and Gallant[10] reviewed 457 breech births and failed to find a significant decrease in mortality or morbidity in the breech fetus born by the cesarean birth route when compared with the vaginal route.

Graves[11] presented data derived from the analysis of breech births between the years 1957 and 1976 in a partnership private practice. In that restricted clinical environment, the fetus below 2500 g appeared to benefit from a cesarean birth. Graves noted equivocal findings for the over 2500-g fetus. He also discussed the impact of the "current torts situation" on physician decision making. Today increased legal risk is an accepted fact of the practicing obstetrician. Thus in the breech presentation, clinical decisions will be influenced not only by what is best for the fetus and mother, but also by which choice poses less risk for the clinician.

In an almost unique prospective study that took place between 1975 and 1979, Collea et al.[12] set stringent management guidelines, including the use of x-ray pelvimetry, and accomplished a randomized trial of vaginal and cesarean birth routes for the frank breech presentation. In their conclusions the authors supported vaginal delivery for term frank breech births and noted that even when the breech presentation in labor was randomized into the cesarean birth route, they could not get all patients to the operating room in time to do the cesarean.

This unresolved debate has continued into the 1990s. Petitti and Golditch[13] described a large private practice group health plan and reported on all birthweights over 1000 g. No demonstrable mortality differences with respect to birth route choice were found. In a study by Bodmer et al.[14] in 1986, the increased cesarean rate did not reduce severe respiratory depression at birth in breech presentation, which is always higher in the breech than in the cephalic presentation. Birth trauma and encephalopathy, when compared with earlier studies, remained the same. The authors cautioned that head entrapment in the under 1000-g population was responsible for 7 deaths of 55 live-born infants, and cesarean was performed least frequently in that population. In a Technical Bulletin produced by the American College of Obstetricians and Gynecologists in 1986,[15] the role of confounding variables was again reviewed, and no firm recommendation regarding birth route given.

Data From the Cleveland Study

Influenced in part by the rising rate of cesarean births in general, and by the preponderance of cesareans for the breech presentation, a retrospective review of breech birth outcomes at Cleveland Metropolitan General Hospital during the 1970s was undertaken to review neurologic morbidity.[16] The study took place in an environment where birth-route choice still existed for the fetus in frank breech presentation. Consultation between patient and physician involved trying to reach a decision as to birth-route choice. Despite the flexibility for birth-route choice in association with this process, more than 60% of breech presentations were delivered by cesarean. The clinical staff was no different in their attitudes toward the breech than the attitudes present in most hospitals.

In the Cleveland retrospective review for neonatal morbidity and mortality, when breech presentations within comparable weight groups were compared, neonatal neurologic morbidity was not decreased by choice for cesarean.[17] When assessing the data within comparable weight groups, it was of interest to note that most breech presentations in labor were born vaginally in the 500- to 750-g category. Above 750 g, the cesarean became the birth route of choice. This implies a new confounding variable that must be considered in the evaluation of all nonrandomized breech studies.

It is apparent that if the physician thinks the fetus is viable, he or she is most likely to treat the fetus differently and this affects outcome. In the Cleveland study, fewer cesareans were performed for the very lowest birthweights when the baby was felt to be nonviable. Thus, if one reviewed overall neonatal risk rather than comparing outcome within small birth categories, the higher incidence of vaginal birth route for low-birthweight fetuses would inevitable bias the review against the vaginal birth route.

Because in the first Cleveland breech study neurologic morbidity was not easily diagnosed before the infants left the nursery, a prospective study was performed to determine infant neurologic outcomes at age 2 years. The vaginally born frank breech presentation was matched by birthweight, with a vaginally born vertex a cesarean born vertex, and a cesarean born breech of similar birthweights.[17] In this quadruple match, major fetal congenital anomalies and in utero fetal deaths prior to arriving at the hospital were excluded. The results confirmed that the morbidity for the frank breech presentation born vaginally was no different than that for the breech born by cesarean of comparable birthweight.

Following both studies, it was clear that morbidity may be influenced by many factors, but the most important factor was the maturity of the fetus.[16,17] While entrapment of the head and prolapse of the umbilical cord did occur, the frequencies of these events were so low and apparently so well recognized (the prolapsed umbilical cord) that these often spoken of fears were not major factors in infant morbidity or mortality. This understanding has led to a philosophy that birth-route choice is acceptable as a treatment option for the fetus in labor as a frank breech presentation. In addition, given the fact that no morbidity differences were apparent at any birthweight, the proposition that cesarean birth is preferred for the very low-birthweight fetus remains undocumented.

Today the birth-route choice controversy continues. More frequently authors consider, on the basis of their findings, vaginal delivery for the frank breech presentation weighing more than 2500 g. Other birthweight windows for cesarean birth often exclude the lowest birthweights on the basis of viability and the over 4000-g fetus on the basis of size.

Based on data obtained from the Cleveland programs, birth-route choice for the frank breech presentation should be presented as an acceptable option for the clinician to offer the patient. This option exists at all birthweights below 4000 g. The Cleveland studies did not have sufficient data to comment on birthweights above 4000 g. In a recent Canadian study, Penkin et al.[18] found that 96% supported a trial of labor for a frank breech presentation and 50% supported a trial for a complete breech.

The Delivery

An Overview

It should be apparent that clinically it is still appropriate to consider vaginal delivery for the frank breech presentation. Yet the clinician should not underestimate nor minimize the potential medical and emotional risks to both patient and physician when considering the vaginal birth route. In the information already presented it was documented that routine use of the cesarean birth route did not avoid all the risks inherent in the frank breech presentation. Birthweight and maturity appeared to be far more important than birth route in infant neurologic outcome,[16,17] and, despite the increased use of the cesarean, decrease in breech presentation morbidity was not apparent.[14] Patient evaluation prior to choosing the birth route, and patient management prior to and during labor, therefore attain prime importance.

Objectives

At the conclusion of this section the clinician should be able to

1. Understand the guidelines for external breech version prior to labor.
2. Present options to the patient for management of the frank breech presentation.
3. Provide management plans for the frank breech presentation prior to labor.
4. Better understand some of the mechanics for frank breech birth.

Evaluation Prior to Labor

The Initial Diagnosis

The initial prenatal visit should be reemphasized as a general approach to all patients. By assessing the patient physically and emotionally during the first visit, including a general appraisal of body size and shape, later decisions can be made with more confidence. A patient 4 ft 10 in. tall is of concern no matter what her fetal presentation is at term. A patient with an abnormal walking gait may have an asymmetrically shaped pelvis. These patients care variables are not as objectively assessed during active labor and are best conducted during early pregnancy. Knowing that a fetus is in breech presentation may alter the clinician's objectivity if pelvimetry and clinical assessment are carried out for the first time.

Information in the antepartum records should describe these initial findings, and an estimate should have been made that a normal-size fetus may traverse the pelvis. In a contrasting example, clinical findings describing a flat or forward sacrum during the patient's first visit will be of major importance during labor. Once the diagnosis of a breech presentation is established and a review of the initial visit suggests limited pelvic capacity, the vaginal route should be avoided and the patient so counseled. There should be no trial of labor in breech presentation in this case. Pelvic capacity is not tested until the fetal head is born. The key thought expressed here is that clinical estimates are assessed prior to the breech position risk. In the presence of the breech, having the information already in place supports a more objective approach.

Patient Emotional State and Patient Involvement in the Decision

Consider the patient's emotional state and her wishes. Some couples come to the physician with outspoken desires for birth-route choice and labor management; others depend on the physician to make the medical decision. There is great diversity. Some patients may be better able to work with physicians during labor and to sustain clinical "crises." Others have more difficulty responding in a constructive way to a difficult labor decision.

EXAMPLE OF PATIENT REQUEST FOR EXTERNAL VERSION

The physician received a phone call from a multipara at 39 weeks of gestation. The caller asked to have an external breech version performed so that a vertex presentation could be obtained. The physician had not seen the patient previously. The patient wished to return to her midwife and deliver vaginally at home. The patient was not reassured by the physician's response over the phone, and she chose to go elsewhere.

Comment

If an external version is performed, the clinician should take responsibility for the vaginal delivery or at least insist that the birth take place in a hospital environment. Often there is a continuum of risk for the breech presentation and preexisting problems incurred prior to labor may be present. The breech, even when turned to a vertex, may represent an already present risk for neurologic maturity. In addition, a return to the breech position following a successful version may occur. The fetus is at risk and should not be considered for a home delivery.

EXAMPLE OF PHYSICIAN BIASING PATIENT CHOICE

A multiparous patient at 39 weeks gestation was told of the frank breech presentation of the fetus and offered a choice of vaginal or abdominal birth. She obtained a second opinion from an obstetrician, who stated that all breech presentations should be delivered by cesarean. She remained with the second obstetrician, who delivered her fetus by cesarean.

Comment

It is evident that on consultation with a second physician, choice was not offered to the patient. It is also apparent that this patient did not wish to make a choice but desired that the obstetrician make the decision. In this example, the offering of a choice for birth route was not acceptable to the patient.

Patient Information

The ground rules for this higher risk situation should be clear. Medical information should be exchanged and discussed when the breech presentation is noted, and the physician should have a chart note documenting the exchange. Should a breech presentation be found first at 30 weeks gestation or at a first early visit, the presentation should be reconfirmed at the next visit. As breech presentation incidence is highest earlier in gestation, it should be reconfirmed at a later visit. If the breech persists, it is time to discuss the facts about breech births and the available options. Although the breech may change to a vertex, the information needs to be discussed at a nonstressful time.

In contrast to the breech presentation found earlier in pregnancy, which usually changes to a vertex presentation during the next several visits, the breech presentation near term should be discussed with the patient when first found. It may, but usually does not, convert to a vertex presentation at or near term.

Although clinical studies suggest that vaginal birth is appropriate, patient choice should be encouraged in this medical situation. If the patient has strong fears or rejects the vaginal route, it is suggested that the clinician should not pursue the issue. The emotional and medicolegal implications are too overwhelming for the physician to be arbitrary.

Antepartum Considerations

Leopold's maneuvers should be performed for all pregnancies at each patient visit after 24 weeks of gestation. If a breech presentation is suspected, ultrasonography should be performed to document the breech and the absence of major congenital anomalies. The breech presentation confirmed prior to labor allows for more discussion with the patient.

The Antepartum Preterm Breech

It is suggested that between 24 and 36 weeks, ultrasonography be ordered at the first detection of the breech presentation. As noted, the breech is more common in incidence early in pregnancy and usually converts to a vertex presentation spontaneously. There is no purpose in alarming the patient. When the breech persists at a second visit, discussions with the patient should begin and ultrasonography should be scheduled. Persistence of the breech presentation for two visits may indicate a reason for the position, rather than a chance occurrence.

The purpose of ultrasonography is to rule out fetal anatomic defects that may be incompatible with life or incompatible with vaginal birth. If a major congenital anomaly is found, or if sufficient time remains, amniocentesis or fetal umbilical cord sampling for the fetal karyotype may document syndromes incompatible with life. These findings would alter the birth-route choice. Umbilical fetal-blood sampling is available in some centers and may be considered if time for karyotyping of amniotic fluid is not available. These vascular studies can be analyzed within days. Fetal karyotype studies are not suggested for the breech-presentation fetus in the absence of morphologic anomalies.

Version of the Term Breech

External Version

From 37 weeks to term, external version should be considered in an attempt to obtain a vertex presentation. More physicians are gaining experience with this technique. Most authors, when reporting on their experience, suggest turning the breech fetus between 36 and 37 weeks.[5,19] As term approaches, increase in fetal size, decrease in amniotic fluid, and lower pelvic position of the breech make version more difficult.

Version Site

External cephalic version should be performed in an environment where a response to unexpected fetal distress during the version may be undertaken rapidly. Umbilical cord problems may be aggravated by the version maneuvers, for example, if the cord is already around a limb or the neck. The use of ultrasonography may allow the clinician to anticipate umbilical cord problems during the procedure. For example, coils of umbilical cord around the neck or limbs may be seen. If bradycardia ensues, the reasons will be clear and the clinical response to discontinue the version will be rapid. Placental separation may occur secondary to the abdominal pressure exerted during the procedure, although this is uncommon. If the patient is Rh-negative, it is possible that sensitization may take place. The use of Rhogam should be considered. Even if Rhogam has already been given at 28 weeks of gestation, additional blocking antibody may be needed if an unusual fetal hemorrhage occurred following the manipulation. There are no data in this area that suggests major fetal hemorrhagic risk.

Uterine Muscle Relaxants

Most version techniques use uterine muscle relaxants such as tocolytics.[5] Some clinicians have used muscle and patient relaxants also. Sufficient amniotic fluid must be present. An external version cannot be performed in the presence of ruptured membranes.

Techniques

Techniques for version are best taught at the bedside, and they are described in standard texts. In general, in the external version one may attempt to turn the head of the fetus forward over its heels. If that does not work, the reverse direction is tried. Constant steady upward pressure is maintained with one hand on the breech elevating it out of the pelvis. At times the breech is so low in the pelvis that the version becomes difficult or impossible. A rotary motion in the direction of the turn is used on the head and back with the other hand. Try to spin the breech around as if following the circumference of a circle. The maternal abdomen should be well lubricated with powder or oil so that the hands move easily in the direction in which the clinician is attempting to turn the breech. This procedure may take 5 to 15 minutes. Ultrasonography should be used at all times during the procedure in order to visualize progress and to follow the fetal heart rate. If unsuccessful in the version, discontinue the procedure. Not all breeches will be turned. Morrison et al,[5] noted reasonable success with an overall lowering of the incidence of breech births at term.

Following the external version, continuous fetal monitoring for the next hour is recommended. Bradycardia of a transient nature often occurs during the version.

EXAMPLE OF THE NEED FOR RULING OUT FETAL DISTRESS

A version of breech to vertex took place without difficulty followed by normal postversion electronic heart-rate monitoring. Later an uncomplicated delivery of the infant in vertex position took place. At 48 hours of age, the neonate convulsed. There was no evidence for an etiology for the convulsion.

Comment

The question persists as to whether neonatal convulsions reflected trauma incurred at the time of the version, or if the trauma was already present in the fetus in the breech presentation. Preexisting breech risk has been described. It was reassuring to the clinician to be able to confirm that no fetal cardiac abnormalities were present during the version or afterwards.

Decisions During Labor

Since it is almost impossible to prepare a patient for every medical possibility and the breech may not be diagnosed until labor onset, discussion about the problems and alternatives of the breech birth take place in a much more difficult environment. In the labor room, faced with the emotions of labor plus an unexpected clinical finding, it is more difficult to offer choices to the patient or family and to have those choices acted upon in an objective manner. Nevertheless, to the greatest extent possible, family consultation is important. The guidelines for care do not change. Discuss and obtain the same kind of permission as would be obtained for any intervention during labor, and record in the patient's chart the fact that the discussion took place and the conclusions that were reached at that time.

EXAMPLE OF UNEXPECTED BREECH PRESENTATION DURING LABOR

A patient was in her fifth pregnancy with a benign past medical and obstetrical history. Labor began 3 hours before arrival at the hospital. A frank breech in LST position at S+1 and full dilatation were found. The estimated fetal size was 7 lb. The patient was beginning to push with each contraction. There was no evidence of fetal distress. She was told of the situation and immediately taken to the delivery room. Thirty-five minutes later she spontaneously vaginally delivered a normal infant over a midline episiotomy.

Comment

A decision had to be made rapidly in a high-tension situation. It was clear that the new findings in labor left little room for an objective patient choice. In this example, the obstetrician assumed responsibility for the medical decision based on the judgment that a normal rapid delivery was anticipated. Unfortunately, someone could argue years later that the 35 minutes of time that elapsed would have enabled the clinician to perform a cesarean. While this may be true, in the prospective management of the breech this could not have been anticipated. This is a time in which the clinician must assume full responsibility, and make a decision based on his or her best medical judgment.

The Hospital Environment

The ability of a hospital to be able to rapidly perform a cesarean for fetal distress or for other unexpected maternal or fetal problems is important. If a management decision is made for a vaginal birth, all support systems for birth route should be in place. Supports include the availability of an operating room, anesthesia support, and the presence of a pediatrician. When these support persons are not available, choices become less flexible.

X-ray Pelvimetry

X-ray pelvimetry has little predictive value. However, even in the presence of a normal pelvis, some will continue to proceed. The logic for a decision to desist from vaginal birth, based on x-ray pelvimetry, cannot be defended any better for the breech than for the vertex. However, noting the many medical and legal pitfalls of the breech birth, it is easier to state to all later questioners that the pelvimetry was normal rather than to defend its absence. If x-ray pelvimetry is not desired or unavailable, depend on the clinical evaluation and careful documentation.

Computed Tomography of the Pelvis

Computed tomography (CT) has been suggested as being useful; and more accurate than x-ray pelvimetry, and it incurs a lower dose of radiation for both breech and vertex presentations.[20] Tomography may demonstrate a better correlation between fetal head size and pelvis, and the measurements may be more accurate. Data on the usefulness of this test, evaluated by controlled clinical studies, are not available. In the end, however, it is usually not size that is the problem of the breech birth, it is the adaptation of the upper body and aftercoming head to the pelvis. Radiography will not likely foreshadow those events.

Intrapartum Care

At the start of labor, a flat film of the abdomen, or preferably an ultrasonography, should be used to demonstrate that the head is not hyperextended. If hyperextended early in labor, the head is more likely to stay in that position during the final phase of delivery. This larger diameter makes for a difficult and potentially traumatic birth. If the head is flexed at the start of the labor, it is less likely to change. In the presence of hyperextension of the fetal head, it is prudent to perform a cesarean. Even with a cesarean, the clinician must be aware of birth mechanics because vertex hyperextension may also lead to a more difficult extraction from the uterus.

Low-BirthWeight Fetus

At all fetal weight estimates, vaginal birth is an acceptable choice for the frank breech presentation. Extraction of a low-birthweight breech from a cesarean incision is also potentially traumatic. Because choice is acceptable at all fetal weights, the problem of estimating size for the small fetus is less important than the question of previability.

Electronic Fetal Monitoring

Perhaps it is unnecessary to state, but for completeness, continuous electronic fetal monitoring is part of the breech surveillance process. The risk of umbilical cord compression, one of the two major risks to the breech in labor (the second is delivery of the aftercoming head), can be recognized and responded to. External monitoring is acceptable if the data are useful. If not, the electrode can be inserted into the fetal buttock.

Pain Medications

Treat a breech birth with pain medications in the same manner as with all other births. If pain medication is needed, analgesia or regional blocks may be used. As with all labor patients, minimal medication and spontaneous birth are preferred. Arguments have been written supporting the use of many forms of medication and regional blocks. No single special medication exists in this area.[21] Individualize patient care and choose the mode of pain relief that the changing circumstances warrant. If the fetus is of low birthweight, concern as to type of medication is more important. Many clinicians prefer to have the patient deliver the fetus spontaneously and without regional block anesthesia, but this is not a universal opinion. Regional blocks can be given that allow the patient to assist in the breech birth.

Oxytocin Use

With each additional complication that may occur, the prudent physician often refrains from vaginal birth and proceeds to cesarean. In the presence of breech birth, the use of oxytocin may be used in the presence of poor contractions or poor progress. In the presence of a normal-size mother and fetus, oxytocin stimulation of labor after spontaneous membrane rupture or augmentation of labor is likewise not contraindicated. However, there is little evidence in any controlled studies supporting a mandated standard of care.

Breech Birth Mechanics

There is no single or best method for delivering the frank breech vaginally. Several general guidelines are suggested.

Anesthesia

In the case of the breech birth, adequate support personnel should be present. An anesthesiologist or anesthetist should be present at the head of the table and be able to administer rapid, complete anesthesia if it is needed. It is important for the patient to know that these events may take place. It is also important to convey to the anesthesiologist that there may be a need for a surgical level of anesthesia with complete muscular and uterine relaxation. Analgesia will not help if a manipulative delivery occurs and the cervix is clamped around the fetal head. All management considerations should be planned ahead with the patient and support staff.

Neonatal Care

Where possible, staff able to provide respiratory support for the neonate should be present. Although respiratory problems are not usual, they should be anticipated. The breech presentation is a high-risk labor, and someone should be available to deliver care to the neonate.

Obstetrical Support

As in a cesarean, when possible, it is helpful to have a second clinician present. That person should palpate the fetal vertex at the start of the delivery and follow it abdominally as it descends into the pelvis and the birth takes place. This individual maintains gentle but continuing pressure on the fetal head in order to maintain flexion and to prevent extension of the aftercoming head as it descends into the pelvis from complicating the birth. As the birth occurs, it may also be necessary to ask for more suprapubic pressure to deliver the head by flexing it into the pelvis if the maternal expulsion efforts are not effective. Knowing where the vertex is at the start and throughout the delivery can facilitate this procedure.

Patience

When the breech is near, the clinician should not interfere. Do not begin to extract the infant or pull it down just because it can be reached and progress is not as rapid as anticipated. Rapid deliveries lead to nuchal arms and extended heads. Listen to the monitor, encourage the mother, be patient, do not intervene.

Episiotomy

As the breech crowns, birth can usually be facilitated by an episiotomy. Performance of a midline incision with the use of local anesthesia is recommended. If necessary, the episiotomy may be extended into the rectum and repaired as a fourth-degree laceration.

Fetal Body Support

As the breech is born, there is a general tendency to extract it. Instead support the breech and the abdomen as the birth progresses. The word *support* is emphasized rather than to *pull*. At the same time, the mother is encouraged to continue to deliver the fetus spontaneously. A spontaneous breech birth with controlled expression of the aftercoming head is always attempted before any intervention.

Umbilical Cord

Many authors suggest that as the abdomen appears the operator should reach up for the umbilical cord and be sure it is pulsating. That is always reassuring; however, the electronic monitor should still be in place. Do not stop monitoring electronically on arrival to the delivery room.

By the time the umbilicus is reached, the cord will be easily available for palpation. It often is difficult for an anxious obstetrician to be certain if it is the cord pulsations that are felt during the delivery or the obstetrician's trembling fingers. However, when the umbilicus is reached, do not expect to delay. The birth should continue to move forward.

Shoulders and Arms

While shoulders may be a problem in a vertex birth, they generally are not the major problem in the breech birth. If spontaneous birth appears slow, traction applied to the body may be needed. When this happens, the development of nuchal arms may occur. The diagnosis is made by a sensation of sudden stopping of descent. By gently placing the hands in the vagina, the arms are seen to be extended above the baby's head, occasionally into the uterus. By gently rotating the infant to one side to gain access to the arm and then by placing the fingers along the fetal humerus, sweeping it down across the infant's face and chest, the arm can be delivered. A repeat procedure can be performed by rotating the infant 180° in the opposite direction. Once nuchal arms occur, further delivery of the infant must be delayed until the arms are delivered to prevent injury to the infant. There is no reason, in a progressing birth, to intervene unless progress has stopped. It is important to allow the aftercoming head to enter the pelvis slowly. If traction is needed, it should be used along with synchronous suprapubic pressure on the fetal head. Traction may be applied from the fetal thighs or presacral region. This is a matter of choice. Some physicians also wrap the infant's body in a towel to facilitate handling.

If only one arm is nuchal and pushing by the mother or gentle body traction does not bring the second arm down, attempt to deliver the nuchal arm with pressure along the humerus. If this is unsuccessful, rotate the fetal body by grasping the free arm and bringing it across the chest. By then the second arm should be down or easily reached.

If attempts to deliver the arms fail, it is time to suspect either an unexpectedly large fetus or poor maternal relaxation. Rapid muscle and uterus relaxing anesthesia is needed. This should have been discussed earlier. This is not a time for analgesia but for surgical level anesthesia.

Aftercoming Head

The major use for the Mauriceau-Smelly-Veight (M-S-V) maneuver is to rotate the aftercoming head into the anteroposterior diameter. The fetal body is still supported, straddled along a supporting arm, and *horizontal* to the floor. In this maneuver some clinicians insert a middle finger into the fetal mouth and place adjacent fingers on the malar eminences to flex the head. Flexion of the fetal head is performed with the M-S-V maneuver. The aftercoming head is more easily flexed by maternal expulsive efforts or by an assistant from the abdominal side. If the head has not delivered spontaneously, now is the time for the assistant to apply suprapubic pressure and to flex the head into the pelvis for delivery.

The delivery of the aftercoming head must be controlled so that birth of the head is not rapidly expulsive. A vaginal hand applied in the M-S-V maneuver can control the birth of the head. Rapid birth of the head results in rapid expansion of the compressed fetal bones and may be traumatic to the dural vessels.

At all times during the delivery, the body is kept horizontal to the floor. Quadriplegia may result from hyperextension resulting from elevating the body above the horizontal or from excessive traction in attempts to flex the aftercoming head through the pelvis. As noted when a problem exists, flexion is best performed from the abdominal side or with the use of Piper forceps.

Piper Forceps

If spontaneous birth has not occurred and suprapubic pressure has not succeeded, proceed without delay to use of the Piper forceps. The application of these forceps is best described in formal texts. However, a few comments will be made about the procedure.

A second attendant is mandatory at this point. This attendant should hold the infant in a horizontal or slightly elevated position to free up the operator for application of the forceps. The blades are applied with the operator kneeling on the floor. If the operator is not low enough, for example, seated on a stool, the position may be too high and the forceps blades cannot be placed alongside the fetal head. The blades are applied in an upward manner following the sacral curve. In a higher seated position, the tendency is to insert the forceps horizontally, which will be obstructed by the sacrum.

One forceps is held by the handle, and the tips of the fingers of the second hand should be placed along the end of the forceps blade. In the vagina, the fetal head will still be felt with the fingertips of one hand while guiding the blade inside the cervix (if it is present) with the other hand. A common Piper forceps application error is to insert the blade under the mandible or the jaw of the fetus, thereby blocking insertion of the forceps blade. This is avoided by feeling for the fetal neck and then the jaw with the fingers placed ahead of the forceps blade. In addition, draw the handle of the forceps toward the midline. This moves the forceps blade away from the midline, and the blade can be felt to go around the mandible and along the head of the fetus. The inserted blade is held by an associate, while the operator is still in the kneeling position and the process is repeated. The blades are locked and traction flexes the head under the pubic symphysis.

Head, Neck, and Body Position

Quadriplegia may arise from hyperextending the fetal head, or following the use of excessive traction on the body of the fetus. Whether born by cesarean or vaginal birth, the fetal body must be kept at or below the horizontal plane of the floor. Do not attempt to flex the fetal head by raising the body above the horizontal. The head cannot be flexed in that manner, and doing so can only incur trauma to the fetal neck.

In delivery by cesarean, this principle also must be kept in mind. Don't elevate the body to ease the head out of the incision. The same damage can occur.

Emotions of Vaginal Breech Birth

By the time one reads through the problems surrounding the breech birth, it is not surprising that cesareans have become so common. The physical and emotional stress to the clinician surrounding the breech birth is duplicated nowhere else in obstetrical patient care. Yet, despite this inner disquiet and the struggle to obtain good data, it is suggested that at all birthweights good clinical judgment allows for a vaginal birth-route choice.

The key points in the process of a breech birth have been described, but this discussion must be considered to be incomplete. The other part of an obstetrician's education is clinical experience, and it should occur at the bedside, hopefully in the presence of a physician who is comfortable with the breech delivery.

Summary

1. Today, the majority of frank breech presentations are delivered by cesarean.

2. The literature documents conflicting opinions based on data for breech births at all birthweights.

3. Confounding variables, important in understanding the literature and in

reaching a clinical birth-route choice in frank breech presentations, include congenital anomalies, prematurity, and preexisting fetal brain damage.

4. At the lowest birthweights, when viability is not expected, most breech births are born vaginally.

5. Despite the increased cesarean birthrate, continuing reduction in infant morbidity is not demonstrated.

6. It is proposed that at all birthweights there is an acceptable argument for birth either vaginally or abdominally, and the choices should be reviewed with the patient prior to reaching a decision.

7. The birth-route choice for the frank breech presentation should be arrived at after discussion with the patient and family whenever possible. Chart notes should document all discussions.

8. Between 24 and 36 weeks of gestation, radiologic or ultrasonographic evaluation of the fetus should take place if the fetal presentation is breech during two consecutive visits.

9. Ultrasonography is used for fetal morphology. Karyotype studies of the fetus should be performed when indicated.

10. In an environment where emergency care may be given, antepartum cephalic version should be attempted near 37 weeks of gestation.

11. Routine radiographic or sonographic review of head position to confirm flexion, monitoring to confirm absence of fetal distress, and pelvic and fetal size evaluation should take place at the start of labor, with the results written in the patient's chart.

12. The labor may be augmented with oxytocin, but in general the need for responding to abnormalities of labor lowers the threshold for choice of cesarean.

13. Analgesia and anesthesia should be available and used as needed.

14. A second obstetrician or other support person should be available for the delivery. A pediatrician or support person for the neonate should be present.

15. The clinician is encouraged, if possible, not to intervene during the birth process; neither pull nor extract the fetus.

16. Piper forceps should be available on the delivery table and applied if spontaneous vertex does not take place.

References

1. Cesarean Childbirth. Bethesda, MD, National Institutes of Health, publication 82-2067. October 1981, pp. 375–386.

2. Brenner WE. Breech presentation. Clin Obstet Gynecol 1978;21:511–513.

3. American College of Obstetricians and Gynecologists. Ultrasound in Pregnancy. ACOG Technical Bulletin 187. Washington, DC, ACOG, 1993

4. Braun FH, Jones KL, Smith DW. Breech presentation as an indicator of fetal abnormality. J Pediatr 1975;86:419–421.

5. Morrison JC, Myatt RE, Martin JN, Jr, et al. External cephalic version of the breech presentation under tocolysis. Am J Obstet Gynecol 1986;154:900–903.

6. Hall JE, Kohl SK, O'Brien F, Ginsberg M. Breech presentation and perinatal mortality. Am J Obstet Gynecol 1965;91:665–683.

7. Berendes HW, Weiss W, Deutschberger J, Jackson E. Factors associated with breech delivery. Am J Public Health 1965;55:708–719.

8. DeCrespigny LJC, Pepperell RJ. Perinatal mortality and morbidity in breech presentation. Obstet Gynecol 1979;53:141–145.

9. Duenholter JH, Wells CE, Reich JS, Santos Ramos R, Jimenez J. A paired controlled study of vaginal and abdominal delivery of the low birth weight breech fetus. Obstet Gynecol 1979;54:310–313.

10. Mann LI, Gallant JM. Modern management of breech delivery. Am J Obstet Gynecol 1979;134:611–614.

11. Graves WK. Breech delivery in twenty years of practice. Am J Obstet Gynecol 1980;137:229–234.

12. Collea JV, Chein C, Quillipn EJ. The randomized management of term frank breech presentation: A study of 208 cases. Am J Obstet Gynecol 1980;137:235–244.

13. Petitti DB, Golditch IM. Mortality in relation to method of delivery in breech infants. Int J Gynecol Obstet 1984;22:189–193.

14. Bodmer B, Benjamin A, McClean FH, Usher PH. Has the use of cesearean section reduced the risks of delivery in the preterm breech presentation? Am J Obstet Gynecol 1986;154:244–250.

15. American College of Obstetricians and Gynecologists. Management of Breech Presentation. ACOG Technical Bulletin 95. Washington, DC, ACOG, 1986.

16. Rosen MG, Chik L. The effect of delivery route on outcome in breech presentation. Am J Obstet Gynecol 1984;148:909–914.

17. Rosen MG, Debanne S, Thompson K, Bilenker RM. Long term neurological morbidity in breech and vertex births. Am J Obstet Gynecol 1985;151:718–720.

18. Penkin P, Cheng M, Hannah M. Survey of Canadian obstetricians regarding the management of term breech presentation. J Obstet Gynecol Can 1996;18:233–243.

19. Zhang J, Bower WA, Fortney JA. Efficacy of external cephalic version: A review. Obstet Gynecol 1993;82:306–312.

20. Federle MP, Cohen HA, Rosenwein M, Brant-Zawadzki MN, Conn CE. Pelvimetry NY digital radiography: A low-dose examination. Radiology 1982;143:733–735.

21. James FM III. Anesthetic considerations for breech or twin delivery. Clin Perinatol 1982;77–94.

Chapter 13

The Third Stage of Labor

Overview

The interval of time from delivery of the infant until the delivery of the placenta is, by definition, the third stage of labor. Most textbooks indicate that this should occur within a period of 15 minutes, while most will occur in a much shorter time. The separation of and expulsion of the placenta is usually accompanied by a sudden gush of blood, concomitant with a descending umbilical cord and a change in the shape and position of the uterus to a globular shape higher in the abdomen.

Objectives

At the conclusion of this chapter, the clinician should

1. Understand the etiology and diagnosis of postpartum hemorrhage as well as suggested management
2. Be able to recognize abnormalities of placental separation
3. Understand the importance of placental examination

Examination of the Postpartum Patient

Once the delivery of the placenta is complete there is a tendency to consider the entire delivery complete. This is an error. An immediate and thorough examination of the vulva, vagina, cervix, and, if indicated, uterine cavity should be undertaken. Hematomas of the vulva or vaginal wall are not uncommon, especially in a prolonged labor, forceps or vacuum delivery, or a rapid descent and expulsion. Examination for the hematoma at this time can spare the patient a painful episode later when the tissues are more edematous. The cervix must be inspected for tears that if present and bleeding, or in excess of 1 cm in length, will need repair. Careful attention to the cervix at this time can prevent difficulty in later pregnancies as well as reduce cervical abnormalities in later life. Should there be any suspicion of uterine tears or retention of parts of the placenta or membranes, an entire uterine examination is indicated. A simple method is to wrap a 4 × 4 gauze sponge around the index and middle finger, insert these fingers into the uterine cavity, and by a gentle rolling motion sweep the sidewalls, the fundus, and the cornual areas.

Examination of the Placenta

Once it has been delivered, the placenta should be examined by the obstetrician before it is removed from the delivery room. Energetic attendants often began cleanup and removal before the obstetrician has completed the examination of the patient and repair of any tears or the episiotomy, if present. This should be guarded against. The cord should be evaluated for length. Does it appear excessively long or short, and if it does what is the measurement? How many vessels does the cord have? Are there knots or other constricted areas in the cord? Are there any missing pieces of the placenta? This can be determined by carefully sponging the maternal surface and observing areas of blood pooling. What is the insertion point of the cord? Do the membranes appear intact?

Finally, is there any gross abnormality or deformity of the placenta? Currently there is debate as to the value of a routine pathologic examination of the placenta. Until further studies are completed, this debate will be unanswerable.

Postpartum Hemorrhage

Following delivery there will usually be a blood loss of 500 to 750 ml. This loss is easily tolerated by the healthy gravida. Therefore, any excess of this amount should be carefully monitored. Since most estimates made at the delivery are grossly inadequate, the rate of blood loss becomes as important as the estimated amount. The clinician should be constantly cognizant of this flow rate. Contrary to many suggestions, most excessive blood loss does not occur in gushes but as a steady stream. The most common etiology is atony, the failure of the uterine muscle to contract sufficiently to close the severed vessels in the placental bed. This is more likely to occur in an over distended uterus, a prolonged labor, in the presence of amnionitis, or with general anesthesia. Careful exploration of the uterus is indicated immediately if lower genital tract bleeding has been eliminated as a cause. If no obvious internal causes, such as uterine rupture or retained placental tissue, are found then massage, compression and oxytocic agents are indicated. Postpartum hemorrhage is one of the most dangerous conditions that women encounter in pregnancy and it must be treated as such.

Failure of Separation

On rare occasions the placenta will not be separated within the usual 15 minute time period. A careful evaluation is indicated to ensure that there is no obstruction to the expulsion, as found in a tightly closed cervix, or that separation has not occurred. If no obvious reason is found, then further waiting is indicated with careful observation of the amount of bleeding and size of the uterus. A large amount of blood can accumulate behind the placenta when it covers the cervical os. Pulling on the umbilical cord to expedite expulsion should be avoided as it has little effect.

If excess bleeding is occurring or the placenta has not been expulsed within 30 minutes, manual removal may be necessary. This is usually accomplished with general anesthesia to prevent severe discomfort to the patient, and this technique is described in most obstetric textbooks.

Example

A gr 4 p 3 has just spontaneously delivered an 8 lb 9 oz infant after a 90 minute labor. There were no complications with the labor, and the infant and mother are bonding well. The placenta has been delivered and the clinician is writing the delivery note when the nurse informs her that there is slow but steady stream of blood coming from the vagina.

Comment

A rapid labor in a multiparous patient should alert the physician to the possibility of postpartum hemorrhage from atony. In this patient a review of the placenta to determine if it is intact and an examination of the vagina and cervix should already have been performed. Assuming no abnormalities were found, the presumptive diagnosis would be atony and appropriate therapy initiated. It is essential that any physician who delivers infants be aware of the myriad of causes of postpartum hemorrhage. This is still one of the leading causes of maternal morbidity in the world.

Other Conditions

Numerous other problems can occur in the immediate postpartum period. It is not the purpose of this book to review them all. Standard obstetrics textbooks give detailed discussions and should be the source of this information. What is essential for the obstetrician is to recognize what is normal and what is abnormal in this stage of labor.

Summary

Management of the third stage of labor can be critical in the gravid patient. A clinician who understands the mechanism of placental separation and the management of the complications is essential to the delivery. After the delivery the clinician should

1. Perform a careful reproductive tract examination, including the uterus cavity if necessary.
2. Be aware of the signs of placental separation and understand how to evaluate nonseparation.
3. Examine the placenta and its attached membrane to evaluate for missing parts or pathology.
4. Carefully observe and record blood loss.
5. Recognize postpartum hemorrhage.

References

1. Diagnosis and Management of Postpartum Hemorrhage. Technical Bulletin #143. Washington, DC, American College of Obstetricians and Gynecologists, July 1990.
2. Placental Pathology. Committee Opinion #125. Washington, DC, American College of Obstetricians and Gynecologists, July 1993.

Chapter 14

Vaginal Birth After Previous Cesarean Delivery

Overview

In the United States, approximately 25% of infants are born by cesarean delivery and about one third of these births is a repeat cesarean delivery. The old dictum of "once a cesarean, always a cesarean" has been refuted by many studies that show *vaginal birth after cesarean delivery* (VBAC) may represent an appropriate option that can result in a decrease in the number of abdominal surgical deliveries.[1] There is a growing consensus among obstetricians that repeat cesarean deliveries should be done for specific indications rather than as part of a routine.

Reports over the last several years indicate that 60% to 80% of trials of labor after a previous cesarean delivery result in successful vaginal births.[2–4] The evaluation of the specific obstetrical history is important in predicting which patients will succeed. For example, women who have previously given birth vaginally and women whose previous cesareans were performed for a non-reassuring heart rate or for breech presentation have higher success rates. Furthermore, even in women for whom the indication for the previous cesarean delivery was "cephalo-pelvic disproportion," up to 70% of these deliver vaginally following a trial of labor. Unfortunately, there is no method that can accurately predict which patients will complete a trial of labor successfully.

Objectives

At the conclusion of this chapter the clinician should

1. Know how to calculate the VBAC rate and the VBAC success rate
2. Identify patients with one or more previous cesarean deliveries who are candidates for a trial of labor
3. Recognize the contraindications to a trial of labor

4. Manage labor and delivery of patients undergoing a trial of labor

5. Assess risks and benefits of a trial of labor

VBAC Definitions

The *VBAC rate,* expressed as a percentage, is defined as the number of VBACs divided by the total number of women with prior cesarean deliveries multiplied by 100.[5] The *VBAC success rate,* expressed as a percentage, is defined as the number of VBACs divided by the number of women who had a trial of labor after cesarean delivery multiplied by 100.[5]

Example

Hospital A delivered a total of 100 patients 100 who had had a previous cesarean delivery in 1995. Of these 100 patients, 50 underwent a trial of labor; 30 of these delivered vaginally.

Hospital B also delivered a total of 100 patients 100 who had had a previous cesarean delivery in 1995. Of these 100 patients, 20 underwent a trial of labor with 16 delivering vaginally.

Question 1. Which institution has the higher VBAC rate?

Question 2. Which institution has the higher VBAC success rate?

Comment

Hospital A has the higher VBAC rate (50/100 × 100 = 50%) compared with hospital B (20/100 × 100 = 20%). On the other hand, hospital B has the higher VBAC success rate (16/20 × 100 = 80%) compared with hospital A (30/50 × 100 = 60%). However, hospital A performs almost twice as many VBACs compared with hospital B (30 compared with 16).

The differences result from the numbers of patients selected to undergo a trial of labor. Often patient preference plays a critical role in the decision to attempt a trial of labor. Despite the relative safety of labor in the presence of a low flap transverse uterine scar, approximately 40% to 50% of women who are eligible for a trial of labor refuse it and instead opt for a repeat cesarean delivery. The most often-cited reasons for this choice are the desire to avoid the pain associated with labor and the convenience of being able to schedule the birth.

Most patients who have had low transverse uterine incisions in previous deliveries are candidates for a trial of labor. This presupposes that they have no contraindications for a vaginal birth. Furthermore, there are data to support a trial of labor in women who have had more than one previous cesarean delivery.[6] The American College of Obstetricians and Gynecologists recommends that women with previous cesarean deliveries be counseled and encouraged to undertake a trial of labor and that this counseling be documented.[7] However, they further recommend that patients not be coerced to undergo either a trial of labor or a repeat cesarean delivery. The patient's decision must ultimately be respected.

Neither is repeat cesarean delivery nor a trial of labor risk free. However, there is evidence that shows that VBAC is associated with shorter hospital stays, fewer postpartum transfusions, and a decreased incidence of postpartum maternal fever.[4] Where reported, perinatal morbidity in this group of patients does not differ significantly from the overall rate at the same institution, and there are studies that report maternal and perinatal mortality rates are not increased in VBAC. However, in a recent study addressing the maternal and perinatal morbidity and mortality associated with a trial of labor in patients with prior cesarean deliveries, major maternal complications were almost twice as likely in the trial of labor group compared with those who underwent a repeat elective cesarean delivery.[8] Most of the serious problems occurred in the group of patients who were finally delivered by cesarean after an unsuccessful trial of labor. The decision to pursue a vaginal delivery should be based on personal preferences as well as statistical outcomes.[9] For the average woman, a successful trial of labor has significant medical advantages, including the avoidance of the hazards of major surgery, and this must be balanced against the slightly increased risk of needing a hysterectomy.

Nevertheless, the most serious risk associated with VBAC is the potential for uterine rupture. Factors associated with uterine rupture include exposure to excessive amounts of oxytocin, dysfunctional labor, and a history of more than one cesarean delivery.[10] But because uterine rupture is potentially life threatening, careful observation of the patient and the ability to perform an emergency cesarean is essential when a trial of labor is allowed. It is best for a trial of labor in a patient with a previous cesarean to be conducted in a hospital environment where these resources are available.

There are a number of contraindications to vaginal birth after a cesarean delivery. Most authorities agree that a previous classical uterine incision has a greater tendency to rupture in a subsequent labor, and patients with a history of a classical incision are not felt to be candidates for a trial of labor. For this reason, generally, if the nature of the previous uterine incision cannot be documented, the patient is most often not considered to be a good candidate for a trial of labor. There are no convincing data on which to make recommendations about how to proceed with patients who have had a lower segment vertical incision as well as previous myomectomy incisions. In these latter two clinical circumstances, if a trial of labor is attempted, one should be prepared to reverse course and to perform a repeat cesarean if any problem arises.

Similarly, there are insufficient data to make strong recommendations about the safety of a trial of labor in patients with uterine scars who have breech presentations, multiple gestations, or fetuses suspected to be in excess of 4000 grams. Although the available studies are frequently too small upon which to draw strong conclusions, in general there does not appear to be an absolute contrandication to conduct carefully observed trials of labor in these clinical situation.

Example

A 31-year-old Asian women has recently immigrated to the United States from mainland China. She has had two full-term pregnancies, both delivered by cesarean in China. She was told that the reason for the cesareans was that the babies were "too big." The medical records are not available. Physical examination reveals a vertical lower abdominal midline scar. She is at term with a singleton pregnancy in a vertex presentation with an estimated fetal weight in excess of 8 lb. The pelvis appears clinically adequate. Contractions have been occurring at 5-minute intervals for a period of 6 hours. On vaginal examination, the vertex is at station –3; the cervix is 4 to 5 cm, dilated, 50% effaced, and the membranes are intact.

Comment

There are a number of issues in this patient that would prompt the obstetrician to approach the decision about a trial of labor with caution. The labor does not appear to be especially effective, and the history of what sounds like cephalo-pelvic disproportion is of concern. Yet neither of these, in and of themselves, would pose a contraindication to a trial of labor. However, the most significant information, or rather lack of information, is the inability to document the specific type of previous uterine incision. The probability that the incision is of the classical variety is high. Therefore, in the patient's best interest, a repeat cesarean delivery should be pursued.

For effective management of patients undergoing a trial of labor after a previous cesarean delivery, each hospital should have the professional and institutional resources to respond to obstetric emergencies. This includes physicians capable of evaluating labor, performing cesarean delivery, and managing the complications of uterine rupture. Patients should be monitored according to the locally established protocols, either by continuous electronic monitoring or by intermittent auscultation. Evaluation of the monitoring tracing or auscultation should take place at least every 5 minutes during the second stage of labor.

There does not appear to be a contraindication to the use of epidural analgesia in the trials of labor in patients with previous cesarean deliveries.[11] Since, most often, the first sign of uterine rupture is a non-reassuring heart-rate pattern or an arrest of labor rather than abdominal pain, the concern about epidural analgesia impairing the ability to diagnose uterine rupture is probably unfounded.

There are differing perspectives on the role the use of oxytocin plays in the management of a trial of labor in patients with previous cesarean deliveries. Some studies show an increase success rate in women who receive augmentation. Paradoxically, there are studies that show an increase in the failure rate among patients in whom oxytocin is utilized. Therefore, this issue remains controversial, and the best recommendation would be to exercise greater caution when administering oxytocin in VBAC trials.

Example

A 25-year-old gravida III, para II was admitted with a history of uterine contractions every 3 to 5 minutes for a period of 2 hours. In the patient's first labor she had a spontaneous delivery of an 8 lb infant without complications. Her second baby was delivered by cesarean because of a transverse lie and weighed 8 lb 4 oz. On physical examination there was a vertex presentation at S = 0 and the cervix was 4 to 5 cm dilated, 90% effaced, and the membranes were ruptured. After an additional 3 hours of observation, the cervical dilatation remained unchanged. The fetal heart pattern was unremarkable and the maternal condition was good.

Comment

This patient's history makes her an excellent candidate for a trial of labor after a previous cesarean because of the prior history of an unremarkable vaginal delivery. For the same reason, because of a failure to progress, and particularly with the vertex at station 0, she is probably a candidate for the judicious use of oxytocin. One can anticipate that she would respond readily and show progression promptly.

Summary

1. Vaginal birth after a cesarean delivery is an appropriate option, and patients with a previous cesarean delivery need to be counseled about the risks and benefits of pursuing a trial of labor.
2. Success rates for VBAC range from 60% to 80%.
3. A previous classical uterine incision is a contraindication for VBAC.

References

1. National Institutes of Health. Cesarean Childbirth. NIH publication no. 82-2067. Washington, DC, U.S. Government Printing Office, 1981, pp. 351–374.
2. Brody CZ, Kosasa TS, Nakayama RT, Hale RW. Vaginal birth after cesarean section in Hawaii. Experience at Kapiolani Medical Center for Women and Children. Hawaii Med J 1993;52:38–42.
3. Cowan RK, Kinch RA, Ellis B, Anderson R. Trial of labor following cesarean delivery. Obstet Gynecol 1994;83:933–936.

4. Flamm BL, Goings JR, Liu Y, Wolde-Tsadik G. Elective repeat cesarean delivery versus trial of labor: A prospective multicenter study. Obstet Gynecol 1994;83: 927–932.

5. ACOG: Committee on Obstetric Practice Opinion. Rate of Vaginal Births After Cesarean Delivery. No. 179. Washington, DC, ACOG, November 1996.

6. Hansell RS, McMurray KB, Huey GR. Vaginal birth after two or more cesarean sections: A five year experience. Birth 1990;17:146–150; discussion 150–151.

7. ACOG: Practice Pattern. Vaginal Delivery After Previous Cesarean Birth. No. 1, Washington, DC, ACOG, August 1995.

8. McMahon MJ, Luther ER, Bowes ER, Olshan AF. Comparison of a trial of labor with an elective second cesarean section. N Engl J Med 1996;335:689–695.

9. Frigoletto, F Jr. Commentary. Natural birth after C-section: The physician's perspective. Health News, October, 1996.

10. Leung AS, Farmer RM, Leung EK, Medearis AL, Paul RH. Risk factors associated with uterine rupture during trial of labor after cesarean delivery: A case control study. Am J Obstet Gynecol 1993;168:1358–1363.

11. Sakala EP, Kaye S, Murray RD, Munson LJ. Epidural analgesia. Effect on the likelihood of a successful trial of labor after cesarean section. J Reprod Med 1990; 35:886–890.

Chapter 15

Informed Consent

Larry P. Griffin, MD, Kenneth V. Heland, JD, and Susannah Jones, JD

Earlier chapters, primarily involving specific phases of obstetrical care, have superficially dealt with the issue of effective communication between a patient and her physician. Nowhere is this more important than in regard to obtaining the informed decision of a patient to choose or to refuse a diagnostic or therapeutic intervention. The issue of whether to inform a patient about significant aspects of her health care has long been resolved. Ethical guidelines of the profession of medicine clearly and explicitly provide that patients have the right to expect and receive such information, and that physicians are ethically obliged to provide it.[1]

In addition, the legal system requires a patient's informed consent to medical treatment or services. A physician who operates on a patient without such consent may be guilty of the crime of battery. Battery is the unlawful or unauthorized touching of another person: *Scholendorff v. Society of New York Hospital,* 211 N.Y. 125, 105 NE 92 (1914); *Canterbury v. Spence,* 464 F.2d 772 (D.C. Cir. 1972); *Mohr v. Williams,* 95 Minn. 261, 104 N.W. 12 (1905); *Perry v. Hodgson,* 168 Ga. 678, 148 S.E. 659 (1929); *Inderbritzen v. Lane Hospital,* 124 Cal. App. 462, 12 P.2d 744 (1932). Lack of informed consent is also an actionable tort in a court of law. The alleged failure to obtain informed consent is at least a compounding factor in up to one third of obstetrics gynecology malpractice cases. This risk is most clearly illustrated in surgical procedures. If a patient experiences an untoward outcome or complication that was not disclosed before the procedure, a court of law could conclude that the patient suffered such a complication due to lack of informed consent. In other words, the court could decide that her physician unfairly manipulated her into accepting a course of action that she would not have taken had she been adequately informed.

Definition of Informed Consent

Although the actual definition from a legal standpoint may vary slightly between jurisdictions, the basic concept is the same. In order for a patient to be adequately informed, and to be capable of giving permission for (consent) or refusing (refusal) a medical intervention, she must be provided with information that permits her to understand the potential and likely benefits. She also needs to know the material risks of both agreeing (consenting) to the intervention and, conversely, of refusing it. In addition she should be made aware of reasonable and appropriate alternate approaches to her condition and their material risks and benefits.

Disputes revolve around the definition of "material" risks and benefits of a procedure and the standard used to evaluate whether this definition was met. Even when such informed consent was obtained, lack of adequate documentation permits questions of fact regarding whether it was properly obtained. This question is often one that can only be answered by a trier of fact in a court of law.

Though many subtle variations are possible, there are two basic definitions of *material* that are applied by courts throughout the country. The first is the *reasonable physician* standard. This standard requires the disclosure to the patient of the risks and benefits that most reasonable physicians believe a patient should know in order to make an informed choice: *Doctors Memorial Hosp. v. Evans,* 543 So. 2d 809 (Fla. App. 1989); *Weekly v. Solomon,* 510 N.E. 2d 152 (Ill. App. 1987); *Davis v. Caldwell,* 445 N.Y.S. 2d 63 (N.Y. 1981).

The second is the *reasonable patient* standard. This standard requires the disclosure to the patient of the risks and benefits that a reasonable patient would expect to know before making a therapeutic choice. The reasonable patient standard is now the rule in a majority of U.S. jurisdictions: *Canterbury v. Spence,* 464 F.2d 772 (D.C. Cir. 1972); *Cobbs v. Grant,* 104 Cal. Rptr. 505 (Cal. 1972); *Halley v. Birbiglia,* 458 N.E. 2d 710 (Mass. 1983); *Festa v. Greenberg,* 511 A.2d 1371 (Pa. Super. 1986).

In both instances, it is agreed that the patient's informed choice must be based on knowledge of the expected benefits, reasonable risks, and appropriate alternatives. In many circumstances, the amount of information disclosed to the patient is the same in the reasonable physician and the reasonable patient standard although the reasonable patient standard usually requires the disclosure of serious but rare complications.

Informed Consent Forms

Physicians and hospitals have often attempted to comply with their informed consent obligation by the use of the *consent form,* which varies in complexity from a blanket consent to all treatment, to forms for specific treatment with complicated explanations of nearly all possible outcomes. Many physicians have felt that a patient's signature on such a form absolves them of any claim of a lack of informed consent. Nothing could be further from the truth.

Though documentation of informed consent is critical, such a form documents only that the patient has seen (not necessarily even read, nor understood) the form.

What is needed is documentation of the informed consent process. Such a process is a dialogue between a patient and her physician, which should not be delegated to someone else. Objective information contained in different forms of patient education materials may help the patient fully understand the issues involved and focus the discussions between the patient and her physician. Such materials, however, do not substitute for the physician–patient dialogue necessary to establish informed consent.

Appropriate documentation should include notes that the discussion occurred, that adequate information on the risks and benefits of the procedure or treatment was provided, and that the patient either accepted or rejected a course of therapy. Such notes should include examples of some significant points covered in the discussion, that the patient seemed to understand, and that questions were addressed appropriately. Any supplemental material provided to the patient should also be noted. Please keep in mind that any third-party educational information made available to your patients in your practice should be reviewed personally by you and a copy retained for future reference.

Informed Consent in Obstetrics

As discussed many times in other parts of this book, there are multiple appropriate options in an uncomplicated obstetrical case. As a result, proper prenatal education is important in order to permit your patients to make informed decisions regarding their health care. Though you are required to present reasonable options, it is permissible and often advisable to make recommendations based on your own training, knowledge, and experience. If the authority of the physician is exercised with respect for the patient's right to reasonable independent judgment, there can be substantial therapeutic benefits. For a physician to present multiple options and then to deny the patient his or her own preference, if one exists, is derelict.

Options such as anesthetic choices, analgesics in labor, etc. should be discussed with the patient during her prenatal course. In all pregnancies, but especially when risk factors are present, discussion in the prenatal course should also include topics such as the use of fetal monitoring, intervention in the event of an emergency in labor, forceps, episiotomy, and other developments that have a reasonable probability of occurring, so that the informed consent process can occur in a non-emergency setting.

It is important that information be presented in a factual way, with balance, and in the form of a dialogue. Following this "educational" part of the process, it is appropriate to express your own recommendations and the basis for them. It is important early in the prenatal course to establish any firm and rigid rules held by either the patient or the physician. In that way, if they are not mutually acceptable, time will permit transfer to another physician. In no circumstances should a physician be compelled to provide treatment he or she considers inappropriate, but such grounds should be agreed upon early in the prenatal course and such an agreement documented.

Informed Consent and Emergencies

In an emergency, it is frequently not possible or practical to provide information to the degree reasonable under non-emergency conditions. Unless your patient is totally incapacitated, she should still be provided with enough information needed to permit her to give informed consent in the context of the emergency. Following resolution of the emergency situation, the therapeutic actions and the basis for them should be explained in depth to the patient.

Informed Consent and Managed Care

With the growth of managed care, additional hurdles can arise in the informed consent process. First, a managed care plan may choose to pay for only one (or less than all) of the reasonable and appropriate methods of management of a condition. This decision might be based on cost "savings." It may also be based on studies that show improved patient outcomes for particular methods of management or treatment. Irrespective of the basis, you are ethically obliged to inform your patients of reasonable alternatives and to have a balanced discussion of risks and benefits. You should inform the patient of the lack of insurance coverage for a particular method of management or treatment so that the patient has information adequate to make an informed choice. This is true despite so-called gag clauses in some managed-care contracts.

Secondly, the reduction in reimbursement for physician services under managed care makes providing lengthy discussions with patients much more difficult. Despite the time and the cost, informed consent is a physician's responsibility. Finally, physicians often feel that if a recommended or chosen course of therapy is denied for coverage by a managed care plan and a complication ensues, the managed care plan is liable. In most cases that is simply not the case.

A physician is expected to be the patient's advocate: *Wickline v. State of California,* 228 Cal. Rptr. 661 (1986). If a recommended treatment is denied, the recommendation and the basis for it should be documented. Additionally, the denial, and your appeal through the established process, should be documented, as should your advice to the patient that despite lack of coverage your recommendation persists.

Informed Consent Tools

As was stated earlier, informed consent forms may be part of the process, but cannot replace it. Recently, the development of the computer-assisted patient interaction has permitted more detailed and individualized approaches to informed consent. One such system, using an interactive touch screen interface, permits the patient to input specific information that allows her to direct the program in a discussion of the material risks and benefits of various ob-gyn procedures and conditions. An individualized printout at the end of the session provides documentation of this interactive informed consent process. In addition, a "doctors' alert" and patient "checklist" serve as tools to focus the face-to-face patient–physician discussion that should follow.

Informed Refusal

Much time has been spent discussing informed consent. It is just as important, however, to document a patient's informed refusal. In effect, what should be documented is informed "choice," whether consent or refusal.[2]

Summary

1. Informed consent is a *process* not a form.
2. *Choice* must be informed and documented, whether it is for consent or refusal.
3. Informed consent is a physician's responsibility.
4. Physicians must serve as patient advocates.
5. Managed care does not relieve a physician of responsibility.
6. Information should began early in and continue throughout the prenatal course.

References

1. American College of Obstetricians and Gynecologists. Ethical Dimensions of Informed Consent. ACOG Committee Opinion 108. Washington, DC, ACOG, 1992.
2. American College of Obstetricians and Gynecologists. Informed Refusal. ACOG Committee Opinion 166. Washington, DC, ACOG, 1995.

Legal Cases

Canterbury v. Spence, 464 F.2d 772 (D.C. Cir. 1972)

Cobbs v. Grant, 104 Cal. Rptr. 505 (Cal. 1972)

Davis v. Caldwell, 445 N.Y.S. 2d 63 (N.Y. 1981)

Doctors Memorial Hosp. v. Evans, 543 So.2d 809 (Fla. App. 1989)

Festa v. Greenberg, 511 A.2d 1371 (Pa. Super. 1986)

Halley v. Birbiglia, 458 N.E. 2d 710 (Mass. 1983)

Inderbritzen v. Lane Hospital, 124 Cal. App. 462, 12 P.2d 744 (1932)

Mohr v. Williams, 95 Minn. 261, 104 N.W. 12 (1905)

Perry v. Hodgson, 168 Ga. 678, 148 S.E. 659 (1929)

Scholendorff v. Society of New York Hospital, 211 N.Y. 125, 105 NE 92 (1914)

Weekly v. Solomon, 510 N.E. 2d 152 (III. App. 1987)

Wickline v. State of California, 228 Cal. Rptr. 661 (1986)

Other References (Books or Treatises)

Appelbaum PS, Lidz CW, and Meisel A. Informed Consent: Legal Theory and Clinical Practice. New York, Oxford University Press, 1987.

Childress JF. Who should decide? Paternalism in Health Care. New York: Oxford University Press, 1982

Faden RR, Beauchamp TL. A History and Theory of Informed Consent. New York, Oxford University Press, 1986.

Rosoff AJ. Informed Consent: A Guide for Health Care Providers. Rockville, MD, Aspen, 1981.

Rosovsky FA. Consent to Treatment: A Practical Guide. Boston, Little, Brown, 1990.

Scully T, Scully C. Playing God: The New World of Medical Choices. New York, Simon & Schuster, 1987.

Chapter 16

Summary of Labor Management

Overview

Today the obstetrician practices in a time when cesarean birthrates have been the subject of increasing public scrutiny. Major reasons for the yearly increase in the cesarean birthrate are the increased numbers of repeat cesarean deliveries, the increased use of the diagnosis of fetal distress, the increased use of the diagnosis of failure to progress, and the increased diagnosis of dystocia. Many of these patient care problems have been presented in this book to assist the clinician in the art of patient care and to urge more consistent patterns of management that encourage vaginal birth.

Objectives

At the conclusion of this chapter, the clinician should

1. Understand the philosophical elements of obstetrical care during labor and delivery.
2. Understand the relationships between obstetrical care and infant neurologic outcome.
3. Be able to make clinical decisions and to weigh the many patient care choices in an orderly manner.
4. Understand the reasons for the rising cesarean birthrate and be able to evaluate the associated patient care decisions in a more critical manner.

Vaginal Birth Following Cesarean

Vaginal birth following cesarean is accepted today by most clinicians as an option, but it is practiced by many with less than full enthusiasm. Vaginal birth following most primary low transverse cesarean sections should be expected and accepted by the physician and patient. Mothers and family members should receive appropriate education early in pregnancy so that the fears of previous labor experiences may be explained or allayed. It is an indication of an obstetrician's attitude and disregard for the data if most of his or her previous cesarean patients are not offered and do not pursue a trial of labor in the next gestation. The data published almost monthly in the literature documents the success of this policy and needs no further verification here.

Fetal Distress

The increased use of the diagnosis of fetal distress is difficult to either explain or justify. In the past 15 years no new information has been learned about heart-rate monitoring and the diagnosis of fetal distress. The criteria for monitoring findings are unchanged, yet, the diagnosis of fetal distress occurs more frequently. It is evident that the diagnosis is being confused. The many pressures existent at the labor scene move the clinician more rapidly to the cesarean birth route. It would appear that the clinician has moved from a diagnosis of fetal distress because of existing data to a "question" or a "possibility" of fetal distress. The treatment of this suspicious zone with cesareans is not likely to lead to any reduction in infant morbidity or mortality but will certainly increase maternal morbidity.

Dystocia

A major portion of this book has been written about the diagnosis of dystocia, which is the basis for a large percentage of primary cesarean births. The use of a language with the same meaning to all is critical. *Dystocia* means different things to different people, so it confuses rather than clarifies. The Friedman nomenclature has withstood the test of time; it is still accurate and allows each clinician to speak in a mutually understood tongue.

With use of the Friedman criteria, given an understanding of what is usual and normal, appropriate treatment programs are available. All too often labors are interrupted without adequate trials. These guidelines are helpful if used.

However, the use of these labor criteria are only guidelines. Arbitrary termination of labor because the labor deviates from the normal curve, or the labor is taking longer than expected, is unacceptable. It is in these situations that the clinician who understands risk and attendant morbidities, and learns to apply judgment rather than to find an excuse for ending the more difficult labors, excels. Patience in following a labor and appropriate nonsurgical interventions in the management of labor are the essence of the practice of obstetrics.

Failure to Progress

Labor usually is a continuous process that progresses in an orderly fashion that can be measured and documented. When this progression is delayed or altered, there is immediate concern. Too often this concern results in an operative delivery for a diagnosis of failure to progress. Recent reports have indicated this diagnosis is occurring with increasing frequency. Whether this is due to earlier recognition of a problem or is just an excuse to perform an operative delivery has not been proven. However, before the diagnosis can be made the clinician must first evaluate all aspects of the labor. This includes fetal position, adequacy of contractions, pelvic measurements, and the physical/emotional status of the patient. Only after these evaluations and corrections of any problems have occurred can the progress of labor be adequately diagnosed. Undiagnosed disproportion, malpresentation, inadequate contractions, or other conditions should not be labeled "failure to progress."

Closing Comments

As stated in the beginning, this text is not designed to give a complete description of labor management and all of its ramifications. It is instead an attempt to propose a plan of management that relies upon the clinician's skills and replaces rote response with reasoned response. Dr. Rosen was a strong advocate of careful documentation, careful evaluation, and response based upon the situation, as it existed. Hopefully, his message has been delivered.

Index